To Leslie

*For your boundless support and
encouragement*

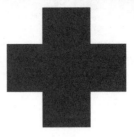

The Emotional First + Aid Kit

A Practical Guide to Life After

Bariatric Surgery

by Cynthia L. Alexander, PsyD

Matrix Medical Communications

The Emotional First + Aid Kit
A Practical Guide to Life After Bariatric Surgery

Copyright © 2006 Matrix Medical Communications

For information address:

Matrix Medical Communications
4975 West Chester Pike
Suite 201
PO Box 445
Edgemont, PA 19028-0445

President/Group Publisher: Robert L. Dougherty
Partner: Patrick Scullin
Executive Editor: Elizabeth A. Klumpp
Associate Editor: Colleen M. Hutchinson
Sales Manager: J. Gregory Francis

Printed in the United States.

ISBN 0-9768526-1-6

Note from the publisher: *This book provides basic information about a broad range of medical conditions. It is not intended to serve as a tool for diagnosing illness, in prescribing treatments, or as a substitute for the physician/patient relationship. All persons concerned about medical symptoms or the possibility of disease are encouraged to seek professional care from an appropriate healthcare provider.*

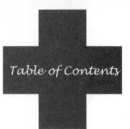

The Emotional First + Aid Kit
*A Practical Guide to Life After
Bariatric Surgery*

- Tune in to Your Own Self-Talk
- Thought Stopping
- Change Negative Self-Talk to More Realistic Self-Talk
- Create a Motivating Visualization

- Default Settings—Our Comfortable Habits
- Healthy Ways to Deal With Stress—28 Ideas
- Progressive Muscle Relaxation Script (PMR)

- What to Say to Yourself
- What to Say to Others
- What to Do
- Mental Rehearsal
- Tips for Attending Parties
- Tips for Eating in Restaurants
- Tips for Navigating the Holidays
- Tips for Cooking for the Family
- Tips for Teenagers

- Self-Talk and Exercise
- Starting the Exercise Program
- "How Much Should I Exercise?"
- "Do I Have to Join a Gym?"
- Exercise Excuses
- Questions to Ask Yourself When Choosing an Exercise Program
- Keeping an Exercise Log
- How to Increase Motivation to Exercise
- The 5-Minute Rule
- Motivation—18 Tips

- Goal Setting
  -Long-term and short-term goals
- Rewards
  -Internal and external rewards

- How to Find Your Eating Triggers
- Behavioral Modification—24 Strategies

- That "In-Between" State
- Seven Great Strategies for Weight Maintenance

- Emergency First Aid

- Sabotage
- Couples Having Surgery Together
- Reminding
- Taking the Easy Way Out
- Family Anger
- Abuse
- Others Concerned With Your Weight

- "When I Look in the Mirror I Am Shocked"
- Feeling Confident
- Feelings of Accomplishment
- Feeling Normal
- Feeling Less Helpless
- Focusing on Other People's Weight
- "My Friends are Jealous of My Weight Loss"
- "I'm Thin, But I Still Feel Different"

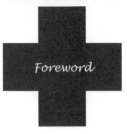

This book's purpose is to help all those wishing to change their lives through bariatric/gastric bypass surgery. As a psychologist, I have seen hundreds of people both before and after surgery and have witnessed firsthand their problems and trials, as well as their successes. In this book, we will discuss many of the difficulties a bariatric patient is likely to encounter and some realistic and practical strategies for dealing with them. Most people go into bariatric surgery full of motivation and hope, only to find day-to-day postoperative existence more stressful than they imagined. Here are the psychological tricks of the trade to help make your own journey a successful one.

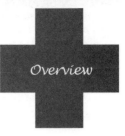

Your Mind is Your Most Important Weapon

I f you are considering bariatric surgery, or have had the surgery, you are facing one of the biggest challenges you will have in your lifetime. Few other decisions will be so life-altering and transformational. The surgery is irreversible, except in the rarest and most dire of circumstances.

Bariatric surgery is often referred to by healthcare providers as a "tool" to help you achieve your weight loss goals. This is an accurate portrayal of the role of bariatric surgery, but many people believe it is much more than that. Many people tend to believe it is the magic pill for which they have been waiting. In reality, life after surgery is very much like living with a very strict diet and exercise plan, just like a traditional diet. All the struggles and temptations that you must master on traditional diet and exercise plans are still there for you to contend with in the years following surgery.

The surgery does not force a person to change. Initially, there will likely be ramifications if the diet is not followed, but eventually those will diminish. Long-term diet and exercise changes are the key to success after surgery, but the surgery will not make these changes happen.

The importance of having realistic expectations cannot be overstated. Those that truly understand what the surgery does and does not provide will have better results.

Many patients come to my office prior to surgery and say, "This surgery will help me because I won't be able to cheat." This is an unrealistic expectation. You can cheat just like on any other diet program. The reality is that most people lose weight for the first six months because it is usually difficult to eat. But just like with a traditional diet, you must watch what you eat and exercise regularly in order to be successful.

It is very important to remember that the surgery component is separate from the lifestyle change component. The lifestyle change involves both regular exercise for life and strict dietary changes. The bonus of the surgery is that you lose weight rapidly if you follow the diet given by the surgeon—the idea being

THE SURGERY DOES NOT FORCE a person to change...Long-term diet and exercise changes are the key to success after surgery, but the surgery will not make these changes happen.

THE BONUS OF THE SURGERY is that you lose weight rapidly if you follow the diet given by the surgeon—the idea being that rapid weight loss will keep you motivated so you will stick with the diet and exercise as you see results.

that rapid weight loss will keep you motivated so you will stick with the diet and exercise as you see results. It will also assist in maintaining the weight loss if you follow the guidelines for life. You will feel full with much less food, and for those with weight-related health problems, such as diabetes, sleep apnea, and high blood pressure, this can be a life-saving surgery.

In this book, I will attempt to provide information acquired over many years in the field of bariatric psychology. Whether you have already had the surgery, are planning to have it, or are still undecided, this information can benefit you in both your weight loss and weight maintenance goals.

In this book, several main themes will be discussed in many different ways and can have great impact on your ability to be successful after surgery:

A. Stress, how it affects your ability to stick with dietary changes and exercise, and what to do about it.
B. How we are our own worst enemy when it comes to lifestyle changes, and how to gain control.
C. Self-talk, what it is, how it works, and how you can use it to help you with eating and exercise.

As you lose weight, you will likely experience many psychological and physical changes. This is your chance at a new beginning, and what that beginning entails is entirely up to you. For some, it means a new wardrobe. For others, it could mean a new career, a new boyfriend or girlfriend, or a chance at a higher quality of life. Even more importantly, it can mean a chance to decrease disease and medication use. The important point is to do what is right for you and for the right reasons. Talk about your situation with friends, family, or a psychologist.

One of my star patients told me she feels as though the day she had her surgery, she was "reborn." She calls herself a "toddler" after having the surgery four years ago. Her rationale is that toddlers have learned much about themselves and their own motivations and still have so much to learn. People who had surgery last month will be learning many new things about themselves every day, much like an infant. She often counsels others to be patient with themselves. After all, it takes many years to unlearn old habits and to get used to the new you. The surgeons agree. I hear them say to patients, "We operate on your stomach, not your head." Bariatric surgery is a wonderful tool, but the rest is up to you.

WHY DO I NEED PSYCHOLOGY AFTER SURGERY?

Many people wonder why psychology is even important. After all, most people will lose a significant amount of weight after surgery. The answer is that psychology helps us to do what we know we should when we have trouble doing it on our own. For example, we all know it is important to eat foods in moderation and to exercise, but do we do it? Of course not. Similarly, after surgery there will be lists of foods you should eat and those you should avoid. There will be suggestions on how often to exercise and lists of vitamins you should take as well. In the beginning, it is easier to follow the set guidelines, but people often struggle with them as time goes on. This is when good psychological tips and techniques can make the difference between success and failure.

The main weapon in your arsenal for weight loss success is your mind. With it, you will learn to change

> ## THE MOST IMPORTANT DIFFERENCE
> between those who are successful and those who regain weight is the proper use of psychology.

the thoughts that keep you from being successful, and use it to establish new habits for life. This time will be different. This time you will not lose the weight just to gain it back again. The most important difference between those who are successful and those who regain weight is the proper use of psychology. If you combine what you learn in this book with the advice of your program's dietitian, surgeon, and others, you will be successful. You will use your mind to change your behaviors and to look at your environment for obstacles to success. Up until now your mind may have worked against you, but starting today, you will be in charge. Starting today, you will begin to learn the techniques and gain the psychological tools that will take you through weight loss and on to weight maintenance for life.

Chapter 1

The Decision to Have Bariatric Surgery

OBJECTIVES
1. Utilize the Pros and Cons Graph in decision making
2. List steps involved in making an informed decision about bariatric surgery

Bariatric surgery itself will vary from program to program and from surgeon to surgeon. There are several different bypass surgeries, and they may be done open or laparoscopically. There are banding procedures as well. While the procedures, risks, and benefits to each one may vary, the lifestyle changes required for long-term success are similar. Each procedure will require long-term dietary changes and exercise for life. The first step is to decide if surgery is right for you.

PROS AND CONS

How do you make a decision that will affect you for the rest of your life? Few decisions you will ever make are as permanent as the decision to have bariatric surgery, much like the decision to have children. Most patients tell me that they agonized over the decision for months or even years before going ahead with it. It is important to look at this realistically in order to make an informed decision. That includes looking closely at all the risks and benefits, including the risk of death, and asking yourself if it is worth that kind of personal risk.

A tried and true psychological method to help make an important decision is to list the pros and cons; therefore, it is a very good idea for patients to list the pros and cons of having the surgery and the pros and cons of not having the surgery. The only catch is that you must be honest and realistic with your answers.

✐ ACTIVITY—THE PROS AND CONS GRAPH

Step 1: On a piece of paper, draw a large box and divide it into four equal squares. Label each box as follows: Pros of having surgery (upper left box); cons of having surgery (upper right box); pros of not having surgery (lower left box); and cons of not having surgery (lower right box) (see page 15).

Now concentrate on one box at a time and make a comprehensive list for each one. Be really honest with yourself, and list everything that comes to mind. It is important to list benefits of not having the surgery, such as less stress, being able to enjoy your favorite celebration rituals involving food, not having to exercise,

Pros of having surgery	*Cons of having surgery*
Pros of not having surgery	*Cons of not having surgery*

etc. Examples of pros for having the surgery are increased mobility and increased self esteem. Take some time to think about this in detail, and write it all down.

Once you have completed this, one box will make more sense to you than the others. It may not be your first choice, but this box may represent the best choice for you.

If your best choice turns out to be to not have the surgery, this may simply mean you really crave weight loss, but are not ready to make the drastic changes that come with bariatric surgery. If this is the case, just wait a few months, and try the pros and cons graph again. Your success with the surgery depends on the dietary

Case Study

Jim came to the hospital using a walker and was barely able to walk down the short hallway to my office. By the time he sat down, he was breathing heavily and was exhausted. He explained that since he had been diagnosed with diabetes and gained the last 50 pounds, his health had steadily deteriorated. It was evident that Jim was finding it difficult to function in his everyday life, and his future looked bleak.

Of course the risks were worrisome to Jim. He said, "It's only going to get worse if I don't do something about this weight." He was unable to exercise due to severe joint pain. He knew he would have to reduce his weight somehow without exercise, and start slowly when his weight decreased to the point when he could move without a walker.

Jim had the surgery, and five months later I saw him at a meeting. He had lost over 100 pounds and was not using a walker. He explained he had started walking and was up to two miles a day. He appeared to be happier, and his health had definitely improved.

Jim's decision to have the surgery was literally to save his life. He told me later the surgery had been a miracle that gave him a "second chance" and that he did not intend to waste that chance.

and exercise changes you must make, so you need to be sure you are committed before deciding to go ahead with the surgery. You only get one chance at success. If you aren't ready to make the lifestyle changes, don't do it.

Other questions you may want to ask yourself:
1. Are the risks and costs worth the benefits?
2. What will I lose if I continue on my present path?
3. Can I honestly say that I have tried my best to lose weight without surgery?

Step 2: Discuss your thoughts and feelings about the surgery with someone you trust. Be sure it is someone who will both listen to your point of view and offer you his or her own opinion. If possible, discuss your decision with several different people who have different viewpoints. It is tempting to just talk to people who will recommend the surgery, but do yourself a favor and talk to people who may be against the surgery as well.

Step 3: Do some research on your own. There is a wealth of information on the Internet and in books. Look at possible complications, the reality of the diet you will be on, and other risks. There are several different procedures available, and each involves risks specific to that procedure. It is important to take a hard and realistic look at the risks involved in the surgery. Candidates tend to discount the risks and emphasize the benefits at this point in the decision-making process.

Step 4: Look at success stories, and talk to as many people as you can that have had the surgery. If you don't know anyone, there are several chatrooms on this topic on the Internet.

Step 5: Discuss your questions and concerns with the surgeon. The surgeon will be affiliated with a hospital-based program. You may request to speak to the dietitian, psychologist, and exercise physiologist with whom the surgeon workds for even more details. Your insurance will probably dictate the facility and surgeon you will use for your surgery. Be sure to check out the surgeon, his or her track record with bariatric surgery, and any complaints that may have been filed against him or her.

Step 6: Take a look at your own weight loss history. Have you been able to reach your weight loss goals with traditional diets, only to then gain it back? If so, then losing weight is not necessarily the problem. Perhaps weight maintenance is your real challenge. Many of my clients tell me they have been unsuccessful at weight loss. In reality, they are very successful at weight loss because they have been able to lose substantial amounts of weight many times, but just need some good solid information on how to maintain that weight loss.

We have been programmed over the years to think of ourselves as either being on a diet or off a diet. Maintaining your weight after weight loss is something in between and requires a whole different mindset. The key to long-term maintenance is exercise. With exercise, you can maintain your goal weight while still enjoying some of your favorite foods. Take a look at your weight loss history. Is it weight loss or is it maintenance following weight loss that is the problem area for you?

If you have come to the conclusion that maintenance is your area of difficulty, then perhaps a healthy diet with the help of appropriate professionals can lead to long-term success. You may wish to consider consulting with a dietitian and a personal trainer or exercise physiologist. See a psychologist to help with those "excuses" we all give ourselves to stop exercising or to cheat on our diets. It may be worth one last try before taking the drastic step of bariatric surgery.

Step 7: Sit down with all of your information and do some honest soul searching. Bariatric surgery can change lives, but it is definitely not for everyone. Once you make a decision, let yourself live with it for a few weeks. With time, you will either feel more comfortable with your decision, or you will have that nagging feeling that you have not made the correct decision. With either choice, you owe it to yourself to take time in choosing whether or not to have the surgery.

Case Study

Jenny could not make a decision about the surgery. Her friends and family were concerned about the risks, but her doctor was recommending the surgery. She had already researched the procedure, spent countless hours thinking about it, and discussed all aspects of the surgery with people she trusted. She decided to make the Pros and Cons Graph, and she was shocked with the results.

She realized that her health would greatly improve with weight loss, and also that she would have to diet and exercise for the rest of her life even with the surgery. She decided to try a healthy diet and exercise plan one more time before having the surgery. All this became clear with the PROS OF NOT HAVING SURGERY box. Jenny said, "I just realized it would be better for me in the long run if I could do this thing without the surgery. I knew my health would improve with any weight loss at all, and it was time to get serious because this is about my health and quality of life. When I really was honest with myself, I realized I didn't want to hear that exercise was important even with the surgery. Once I accepted that exercise was required with or without the surgery, I just decided to give it another shot."

For Jenny it took a couple of difficult months to really get into her new program, but after three months she had developed many new healthy habits. Both a personal trainer and dietitian were consulted during the initial weeks. She began exercising four times per week, and made many changes in her eating patterns. Jenny lost 36 pounds in three months, and has been steadily losing ever since.

Of course Jenny still had options. She was young and did not yet have any of the health problems associated with obesity. Many people are not this lucky.

The choice to have the surgery should be made with your doctors and people you trust. Some patients become glowing success stories, while others fall back into old habits and never realize their weight loss goals.

Chapter 2

How to Prepare Yourself Psychologically Before Surgery

OBJECTIVES

1. Differentiate between lifestyle changes (recreational eating, exercise, and emotional eating) and surgery (pouch)
2. Describe the SAFE ZONE
3. Identify questions to discuss with family members prior to surgery
4. Complete the Emotional Situations Eating Form
5. Contrast real and emotional hunger
6. Construct a list of activities that will substitute for emotional/recreational eating

There are many things you can do prior to surgery to prepare yourself, and all of these will increase your chances of success after surgery. Start the changes as far ahead of the surgery as possible. Shoot for at least 6 to 8 weeks before your scheduled surgery date.

The six main areas of preparation, which are all covered in more detail, are as follows:

1. Prepare your environment.
2. Prepare your support system.
3. Emphasize the activity rather than the food.
4. Learn to structure your eating pattern.
5. Control emotional eating/recreational eating.
6. Begin a consistent exercise routine.

WHY SHOULD I PREPARE BEFORE SURGERY?

Think of bariatric surgery as consisting of two entirely separate components: 1) the surgery itself—the creation of the pouch; and 2) the lifestyle changes. These lifestyle changes include stopping the emotional/recreational eating and maintaining a consistent exercise routine.

There seems to be an expectation that the surgery itself will force the lifestyle changes that must follow, but this is not the case. For the first 3 to 6 months, the surgery will make it easier to change your diet. For example, you may get sick or feel uncomfortable if you eat too much, eat the wrong foods, or do not chew enough, but after that initial period, it becomes mind over matter. The surgery will not force you to exercise or change your recreational or emotional eating habits. To successfully make all the necessary lifestyle changes, you will rely heavily on using your mind for adherence.

Lifestyle changes must last for life. This sounds simple, but how many times have you made lifestyle changes in the past, only to fall right back into those old eating patterns when you were bored, went through stress or changes at work, or went to a party and "blew it?" It is normal to fall off the wagon, but this time you can learn to use your mind to keep from going down that same road. The mind dictates your ability to stick with lifestyle changes, and this time it has to be for the rest of your life.

Case Study

Margaret always had a sweet tooth. Thinking of her husband, she bought his favorite candy bars and ice cream every time she went grocery shopping. Coincidentally these were also her favorite candy bars and ice cream. When she was tired or bored, her resolve to stick to her diet seemed to disappear, and she often ate some of the treats that were in the house "for her husband."

There was always a full candy jar on her desk at work "for other people," but she was most often the one to indulge.

She seemed to plateau early in her weight loss. The nurse at the surgeon's office inquired about her eating habits. Margaret was confronted on the need to have her favorite foods in the house, and she conceded she was having great difficulty giving up her lifelong comfort foods.

Margaret agreed not to bring these items into the house again, and decided that her husband could get ice cream or candy bars himself if he so desired. The candy jar on her desk had to go, too. Through this experience, she began to understand the power of the mind in helping or hindering her in dietary adherence.

When Margaret was weighed the next month she had lost 15 pounds, and had more control over her eating habits. She said, "I always had a really good excuse for keeping the food around, but now I understand these excuses keep me from achieving my goals."

OUTDATED THINKING

Remember that lifestyle changes are separate from the surgery. Most people combine the two components in their minds, saying, "When I have the surgery, I will have to change my life." This is an example of outdated thinking when it comes to bariatric surgery. The old thinking is to wait for the surgery to start the lifestyle changes. The new thinking is to start the lifestyle changes as far ahead of the surgery as possible. This will give you more confidence and also give you a jump start on the long road ahead.

The best advice you will get is to establish all of your healthy habits prior to surgery. The last piece of the puzzle is the surgery itself. The most difficult part of the process is the lifestyle change, and if you master this before the surgery, you will do much better and have much less stress. By the time you add the final step of surgery, you are already on the road to better health. Patients who have prepared in this way report that it has been a positive experience.

> **THE BEST ADVICE YOU WILL GET** is to establish all of your healthy habits prior to surgery. The last piece of the puzzle is the surgery itself.

Many people like to have "last meals" before the surgery. This is expected, but a much better use of your time is getting into all of the habits you must follow after the operation. Changing your lifestyle is difficult under the best circumstances, but after surgery when you may be tired, irritable, and sore from the procedure, it will be much more difficult.

PREPARING YOUR HOME ENVIRONMENT

How many times have you said to yourself, "I didn't plan to eat the ice cream, but it was in the house and I had a moment of weakness?" Anyone who has ever attempted to change eating patterns can relate to this. The solution to this problem is to make sure you do not have foods in the house that will tempt you. It is imperative that you turn your home into a bariatric-friendly environment.

How do you make your home bariatric-friendly? The key is to remove all trigger foods. Everyone has several foods that call to them from the refrigerator or the cabinet. It will be next to impossible to stay true to your bariatric diet if these foods remain in your home. After a hard day at the office or a personal crisis, it is very difficult to resist these foods. During a moment of weakness or hunger it is easy to eat the food, then immediately regret it. I hear this complaint from patients even years after surgery. Somehow those foods find their way back into the house, at about the same time willpower slips out the window. The first line of defense is to take all these foods out of your home. It is hard to do, but it is time to live your life without them.

WILLPOWER DOES NOT ALWAYS WORK

This is a difficult transition, but necessary if you are to achieve your weight loss goals. Trigger foods must be removed from the home. This is NOT an option. Trigger foods are the ones that we will eat if they are in the house. They are the foods we usually choose when we cheat. Everyone has a few of these. If they are present, it will be much more difficult to stick to your diet. Compare it to a person who is trying to quit smoking. If there are cigarettes in the house, and others are smoking, it will be next to impossible to quit. How about the alcoholic who thinks he can meet his friends in a bar, but will just drink milk? Not very realistic, and he is putting himself in a situation where he will have to rely on sheer willpower. Willpower is not consistent, so the goal is to eliminate it as a variable in your weight loss. Set up your environment for success. Begin to create a bariatric-friendly environment.

Become aware of roadblocks to success. Like a detective, scrutinize your environment, your home, your work environment, and your habits for obstacles. The goal is to completely take willpower out of the equation. When we rely on willpower, we are more likely to lose the battle. Don't put yourself in a situation where you have to rely on willpower until you know you can handle it.

Be aware of the kinds of thoughts that entice us to bring certain foods into the house. If you think you must have sweets or some other non-bariatric food around for your family, then be certain to buy the items you don't like. Is it coincidence that when we bring treats into the house for "other people," these are our favorite treats as well? What are the chances we can resist these foods when under stress, or when having a bad day, or having a craving? If you need an incentive, tell yourself your kids can live without cookies for a while and will probably learn some very healthy eating habits in the process.

When you reach your goal weight, you can do a little test. Try your trigger foods. If you are able to eat appropriate amounts, you may consider adding small amounts back into your diet. If you find you feel out of control with the foods, or are unable to regulate the amounts, then you may end up having to trade that trigger food for good health. Don't try this experiment until you've already reached your goal weight.

CREATE A SAFE ZONE

Create a SAFE ZONE in your home by promising yourself not to bring in anything tempting or off your

Case Study

Dave knew before the surgery that his family was going to be trouble for him. Whenever he brought up the lifestyle changes he would have to make after surgery, his two teenage sons would say, "I hope you don't expect me to eat like you do."

He realized that if his family members were divided, it would be difficult for him to stick to the diet. Teenage boys tend to eat more, and often bring junk food into the house. He knew the temptation at home was likely to be overwhelming for him. He also realized that his boys had learned some poor eating habits from him over the years, and he saw this as an opportunity to help them change these habits.

Dave called a family meeting and openly discussed his concerns and hopes for his sons. The boys listened, and could see this was important to their father and likely to benefit them also. He made it clear that they would all benefit physically, and they would have more high quality time with Dad because he would have the energy and mobility to engage in activities with them. He let them know that there was something to be gained for them as well. This was helpful as the boys did keep tempting foods out of the house. The last I heard they took a bicycling vacation together and had a wonderful time.

diet, regardless of the quality of the excuse. It is much more difficult to cheat if you have to leave your home to do it, and there are plenty of chances to talk yourself out of it on the way to the store. Imagine how much easier it will be to adhere to the dietary guidelines when you walk in your front door after work and can let down your guard. You won't have to worry about willpower or cheating. You don't need it because you are in a SAFE ZONE. In your safe zone are plenty of bariatric-friendly foods, snacks, and drinks, but no trigger foods.

Remember, you do not want to rely on willpower to keep you on track, but rather an environment designed for bariatric success. This strategy boosts your chances of success, and is one of the most basic rules.

PREPARING YOUR SUPPORT SYSTEM

The people in your life will have an effect on your ability to stick with the lifestyle changes you must make. You will need to prepare them for changes they can expect, and to let them know the important role that they will play in your weight loss journey. Supportive family members will make it easier for you, and non-supportive family members can wreak havoc with your diet and your resolve to eat properly. Keep in mind that it is very difficult for family members during this process as well.

If you live with other people, it makes sense to discuss with them the impending changes you will be making. I like to have whole families commit to using this as an opportunity to become healthier. Discuss any areas of concern with everyone living in the house as far ahead of the surgery as possible. If you approach your family with a coherent plan, they will be more receptive. Here are 11 questions to ask yourself:

1. How will meals change in the home?
2. What foods will and will not be available in the home? Discuss the concept of the SAFE ZONE.
3. How will the family benefit from you being healthier?
4. What can the family members do to help you be successful?
5. How should family members handle the situation if they decide to eat something they know will be tempting for you?

6. How will you handle having guests in the home?
7. How would the family like you to handle your new diet?
8. How will you deal with holidays and parties in the home?
9. Would your family like to use this as an opportunity to be healthier and more active themselves? If so, how can you all motivate and support each other?
10. Tell your family what to expect in the days and weeks after surgery. Explain the hospital stay and how you will need help completing some tasks for a while.
11. The radical dietary changes usually last about one year and then you are able to eat more normally, just with smaller portions. It often helps to let the family know there is a light at the end of the tunnel.

SUPPORTIVE FAMILY MEMBERS will make it easier for you, and non-supportive family members can wreak havoc with your diet and your resolve to eat properly.

Making sure that your family members are involved in the decision process will make it easier for everyone. If you are living alone, the changes will be a little easier for you. Often family members are resistant to change because they are not the ones deciding to do this.

Make sure everyone in the family understands how this can benefit them, from losing weight themselves to doing more activities together. When you become healthier and lose weight, others will also reap the rewards.

RECREATIONAL AND EMOTIONAL EATING

It is very common to hear, "If I could just find out why I eat this way, it would be so easy to stop." Some people want to figure out why they eat for emotional reasons. The fact is, you don't need to know why in order to change. Even if you are able to get to the root of your emotional eating, that information will not usually automatically lead to change. It may be helpful to know why, and you may be very curious, but that knowledge is not of key importance to your weight loss. For most people, it makes sense to skip this quest, and proceed directly to the step of changing the habit. It is important to look at the emotions you experience when feeling out of control, but it may not be necessary to find the root of the problem in the past.

Eating for emotional and recreational reasons is very common. Everyone does it to some extent, but giving in to that will make it very difficult to achieve lasting weight loss. You can prepare yourself to deal with those thoughts and situations so that food doesn't run your life.

Expect to always feel conflict about eating. Except for the first few months after surgery, you will probably want to go back to eating your favorite foods. If you expect the conflict, you can plan to deal with it and win the battle of recreational and emotional eating. In the beginning, most people will experience a decrease in hunger and cravings. This is called the "honeymoon period." It's easy to stick to the dietary regimen because you are simply not hungry.

The shock for many patients is that when the hunger returns, the cravings and thoughts of food do, too. For a small percentage, they will never lose the cravings, and must battle the urges right after surgery. I have some patients that had the surgery four or five years ago, and they tell me it is still a daily struggle to remain true to a healthy diet. The hard truth is that if you use food for comfort or other emotional reasons, those thoughts and cravings will probably always be there. Once the connections are established between food and emotions, they will not easily go away. They may diminish in intensity with time, but will likely be a part of your life for a very long time.

> **SOME PEOPLE WANT TO FIGURE OUT** why they eat for emotional reasons. The fact is, you don't need to know why in order to change.

Before surgery you can begin to experiment with eating only your planned meals and snacks, and when you crave food at other times there are some things you can do. Start by keeping yourself busy, by taking yourself out of the situation, or by figuring out why you want to eat and finding another way to satisfy the need. Here is an example: You would normally eat to reduce anxiety, but instead of eating, try spending time on the phone with a friend or taking a hot bath. If you start to do this before the surgery, you will find several alternatives that work. This will give you confidence and prepare you for those same situations after surgery.

We eat because we are hungry and for a host of other reasons. Some common traditions and stressors that cause people to eat are family get-togethers and holidays or out of habit, anger, sadness, stress, and boredom. Or we create excuses for ourselves to make it acceptable, such as "It's Friday," "I'm celebrating," "I have to have wings because the game is on," or "I can't enjoy the movie without popcorn." You may not be hungry when you go to the family picnic, but when you get a familiar whiff of Aunt Betty's famous apple pie, you will want to eat it. This type of conflict will not go away, and it is the cause of much stress for the bariatric patient. You will gain confidence and control with experience, but expect to always have the cravings to some degree. One of my patients asked in reference to her love of food, "Will I ever get this monkey off my back?" The short answer is no. It will become a smaller monkey, and you will have much more control over it, but you should expect it to always be there to some extent. The monkey may become dormant, but it can come to life with stressful events or major changes in your life.

✐ ACTIVITY

Begin to look at all the situations in which you eat. Listing them is very helpful. Rate each one on a scale of 1 to 10 (with 10 being the most difficult to control).

Common reasons that show up on these lists are going out to dinner or a movie, holiday parties, sporting events, boredom, loneliness, sadness, celebration, or television viewing.

Try to set up your schedule and environment so they do not dictate whether or not you eat certain

	M	T	W	Th	F	Sat	Sun
Time							
Food							
Emotion before eating							
Unusual circum-stances							

Sample Emotional Eating Situations Form
Visit www.bariatrictimes.com for a downloadable PDF of this graph.

foods. Try not to put yourself in any situation you rated 6 through 10 until you know you are ready.

To use the Emotional Eating Situations Form, record the date, time of day, day of the week, the food you consumed, your emotion just before eating, and the circumstances at that time. After a few days, you will have a good idea of what emotions lead you to eat and you will understand how to intervene. For example, if you most often eat when bored, then perhaps starting various projects around the house, taking up a new hobby, or going to the movies will keep you from eating out of boredom. If you eat because you are lonely, then perhaps calling a friend or relative or visiting someone you haven't seen in awhile will be helpful.

Even though recreational eating is normal, it is something you should not do after surgery. Chances are you've been on many diets in the past if you are considering bariatric surgery, and you know how difficult it is to sustain strict dietary changes over time. Expect to always have conflict between the thoughts, "I really, really want to eat this," and "I know I shouldn't." Don't expect to magically not want to eat or be given some incredible willpower that you haven't had in the past. It is still possible to overindulge, and it is an all too common occurrence for people who have unrealistic expectations of the surgery.

Many people believe the surgery will prevent them from overeating, and they are both right and wrong. During the first few weeks after surgery, it will be almost impossible to overeat. You will be on a liquid

> **THE MOST POWERFUL WEAPON** to help you resist eating for life is not the pouch, but the mind.

diet, and food may not look very appetizing. It is when solid food is reintroduced into your diet that you must be careful. This usually occurs a few weeks after the surgery. Once you are able to eat again, you will probably crave your favorite foods. It will be a challenge to resist, just as it has been in the past. People tell me, "I won't eat the foods I'm not supposed to eat after surgery because it will make me sick." Unfortunately some people will try eating their favorite foods anyway, only to find they don't get sick.

Consider the person who is on a diabetic diet and does not follow it. The consequences can be severe, but it does not stop people from cheating. The same is true of the surgery. Many patients think, "This will really stop me from overeating. This time I will have to do what I am supposed to do." Or, "Why would I eat the wrong foods when I risked my life for this surgery?" Or, "I'll get sick if I eat the wrong foods." This may sustain you for the short term, but don't count on it for the long term. The surgery will assist you, but it is still your decision whether you will cheat or whether you will stick with your bariatric diet. Like the person who is not following his or her prescribed diabetic diet, people will cheat with this diet, too. The most powerful weapon to help you resist eating for life is not the pouch, but the mind.

REAL OR EMOTIONAL HUNGER?

For the new bariatric patient, you will most likely not feel true hunger for several months. It is important to eat as directed even when you might not be physically hungry. But for those starting these changes prior to surgery, or whose hunger has returned after surgery, it is important to distinguish between true hunger and head hunger.

True hunger, or physiological hunger, involves hunger pangs, stomach growling, or feeling weak or shaky from lack of food. This is the hunger that requires the response of eating. Over the years, many people lose the ability to recognize real hunger or differentiate between real and emotional hunger.

"Head hunger," or emotional hunger, must be controlled in order to be successful with long-term weight loss and maintenance. When you eat in response to a situation, like a holiday party or the smell of food cooking, or for emotional reasons, like stress or loneliness, you are responding to head hunger.

Ask yourself when you eat, "Is this true hunger or is this head hunger?" If the answer is head hunger, then it is time to change your environment, thoughts, activities, or situation. First take yourself out of the situation. Leave the kitchen, turn off the TV, or go outside and take a breath of fresh air. Take a short time-out to gain control, and then say something motivating to yourself, such as, "This is about my health, not food. I can do this."

Now that you have a realistic view of what to expect after surgery, imagine going to your first holiday party. Perhaps you had the operation four months prior and are feeling very confident. What will your strategy be? What will your escape plan be

DON'T WAIT UNTIL YOU are at your goal weight to begin enjoying those activities you have always dreamed of doing once you lost weight. Start now and it will be easier to stick to the diet because you are already enjoying yourself more.

if you begin to feel overwhelmed? What will you say to people? Plan all of this ahead of time for your best chance of success. Remember you will likely want to eat. Expect to have that conflict between wanting to eat and wanting to stick to the diet. Do not expect it to be easy for you. You may feel like you are on the outside looking in. It will get easier with time, but it will take multiple exposures to these types of situations to increase your confidence and your ability to stick to your plan.

BEGINNING THE FOOD EMPHASIS SHIFT

It is helpful to begin to think of food as fuel and your body as a work in progress. Every day will bring you closer to your goal as you lose a few more ounces and gain strength through exercise. Keep your eye on weight loss, improving health, and your long-term goals.

Food has been a "best friend" for some. If this is the case for you, there will be additional challenges. They don't call it "comfort food" for nothing. During times of stress, your thoughts may automatically turn to food, and you will have to override some pretty intense feelings in order to stick with your diet. I always suggest people write down when and why they eat. Are you really hungry? Or are you bored? Keep a list handy of alternatives to keep you busy, and call a friend if necessary. Get yourself away from the temptation, whatever it may be. My patients tell me they do well when they anticipate that changing habits will be difficult. Those that think it will be easy or automatic usually have a more difficult time.

Take steps to shift the emphasis from what you are eating to what you are doing. For example, instead of planning dinner out for Saturday night, think about the movie you will see or a trip to the beach to watch the moon rise. Most people dream of the exciting activities they will do when they lose weight. This is the time to think about and try those activities because it will give you power over eating and provide the motivation you need. Over time food will become secondary and will lose some of the hold it may have on your life. Don't wait until you are at your goal weight to begin enjoying those activities. Start now and it will be easier to stick to the diet because you are already enjoying yourself more.

✓ TO DO

Make a list of activities you can do instead of eating. When an urge to eat occurs, try one of the activities on your list. Keep the activities that work for you and discard those that don't. Another idea is to schedule your daily exercise during that time of day you are most likely to overindulge. Make sure your plan is realistic. It is not reasonable to expect to exercise every time you feel like eating. Some other positive

THESE CHANGES SEEM SIMPLE, but even retraining your automatic eating pattern requires concentration.

activities could be to call a friend, take the dog for a walk, surf the Internet, have a glass of water, watch a movie, read a book, get involved in a hobby or craft, and on occasion exercise. Of course you will still be able to eat, but shifting the emphasis to activity will help with the psychological transition.

STRUCTURED EATING PATTERN

Start some food changes a couple of months ahead of your surgery. Keep in mind that these lifestyle changes are entirely separate from the surgery, and everything you do ahead of surgery will lead to greater chances of long-term success. Start to structure your eating pattern. Have three healthy main meals and a couple of healthy planned snacks if you need them. Be prepared and shop ahead. If you take your healthy foods to work, it will go a long way to eliminate the desire for fast food, vending machine snacks, etc. This will prepare you for life after surgery. Getting into the habit of always having healthy foods with you and avoiding the old habits will help make an easier transition.

You may also experiment with some of the bariatric foods you will be required to eat after surgery, and start teaching yourself how to chew each bite of food 25 to 30 times before swallowing. Begin training yourself to always have a bottle of water with you. Try to get in the habit of stopping drinking well before meal time and starting at least 30 minutes after you eat. You will be instructed to do this after the surgery, so trying to develop those new patterns in advance will only serve to help you later. These changes seem simple, but even retraining your automatic eating pattern requires concentration. It will take some time to become comfortable with not swallowing after just a few bites.

Chapter 3

Self-Talk

OBJECTIVES

1. Differentiate between positive and negative self-talk
2. Explain how self-talk influences motivation to exercise, or adhere to the bariatric diet
3. List positive motivating phrases that can be used to increase motivation
4. Practice deep breathing to decrease anxiety
5. Use the Thought Stopping technique to stop negative, self-defeating thoughts
6. Construct a motivating visual of you at your goal weight

An important question that comes up when trying to adjust to lifestyle changes is "How do we overcome a lifetime of recreational and emotional eating?" Part of the answer is in the concept of SELF-TALK.

A very important key to your success following surgery is your ability to control your own self-talk. Self-talk is what goes on inside your head automatically. What you say to yourself will either put you in control of your life or give you a passive role in your own health and success after surgery. Controlling your self-talk is key to dietary and exercise adherence after surgery. Self-talk is discussed in many different contexts in this book, as follows:

- Using self-talk to increase motivation to exercise
- Using self-talk to control emotional eating
- Using self-talk for long-term weight maintenance.

Self-talk determines if you give in to eating the cheeseburger or say no and have the chicken breast. Self-talk determines if you skip your workout or go outside and walk for 30 minutes. Self-talk determines if you feel positive or negative about the surgery and your progress. Self-talk determines if you eat cookies because you are depressed or pick up the phone and call a friend instead. Self-talk plays a large part in life after bariatric surgery, and for many, it can ultimately determine success or failure.

Most people are unaware of the conversation that goes on inside their own heads all day, every day and are, therefore, unaware of the great effect it has on how they feel and act. In order to control your self-talk, you must first become aware of its existence. Let's look at some examples.

✐ ACTIVITY

Self-talk is not necessarily what we say out loud, but what we think and say to ourselves inside our heads. Test: Try saying something positive to yourself, and you will find that you instantly feel better than when you say something negative to

> ## *Tip*
> Think of your mind as a radio, and you control the
> radio stations. You can turn the channel from negative
> self-talk to a channel with positive self-talk. Remember,
> you have the ultimate control over your thoughts. They
> do not control you unless you allow them.

yourself. For example, say, "This is going to be a good
day." You will feel better than if you say, "Here comes
another terrible day."

This internal dialogue takes place constantly, but
most of us are not even aware of it and operate on
"automatic." Think back to when you learned a new
skill, such as using a computer, riding a bicycle, or
playing a sport. If you said to yourself, "This is fun. I
know I can do it," chances are you did. If you said to
yourself, "I'll never be able to do this," chances are
you had difficulty. I talk to people who say, "I don't
have self-talk. I just am the way I am." Everyone has
self-talk and can learn to control it. It's just a matter
of learning to recognize it.

Professional golfers and other athletes understand
the power of the mind when it comes to success.
There are psychologists who work exclusively with
athletes to help them use these techniques to gain
control of their behavior, reduce anxiety, increase
confidence, and control the powerful messages of the
mind. The messages you give yourself every day will
have an impact on your ability to succeed in weight
loss after surgery.

SELF-TALK: LISTENING TO THE EXCUSES

When it comes to diets, self-talk can determine
success or failure. People start diets full of hope and

motivation, but often that determination disappears by the third or fourth day. The culprit is usually self-defeating self-talk. How many times have you been on a diet and said to yourself, "I deserve a treat. I've been good all day." Before you know it, you've eaten something you did not plan to eat. Or how about when you say, "I'll just eat a little bit less tomorrow to make up for it." At that point you have eaten too many calories for the day and may just decide to keep on going. The self-talk usually goes something like, "I've already blown it today, so I'll just start again tomorrow." The next day you find your motivation has greatly decreased, and you may cheat again. By the following day you are off the diet completely. The next usual step is to say, "I'll just start again Monday," but when Monday arrives, your motivation has completely disappeared.

If this same person had said to herself, "If I exercise for 45 minutes today, THEN I can have that treat," or "I don't need that treat because this diet is about my feeling better and looking better," she might not have cheated.

A THEORY

Evolutionary psychologists have a theory. Human beings have been around for many thousands of years. For most of the history of our human existence, food was scarce and we learned to eat whenever possible. With the exception of the last few hundred years, people often did not know when they might be able to consume another meal. When it comes to exercise, conserving energy was a priority of our past because we needed energy to be available to fight, work, farm, or travel long distances. Things have changed radically. In the last few generations,

calorie-dense, high-fat food has become abundant,
and there is very little need in the lives of modern
human beings to expend large amounts of energy.
The result is that now we need to restrict our food
intake and force ourselves to exercise to maintain a
healthy weight.

If this theory makes sense, then you may agree
with what happens next. Since "dieting" or "working
out" are relatively new concepts for human beings, it
is as if we are going against our own instincts. Then
something very interesting happens. Our minds begin
to work against us, too. We actually become our own
worst enemy. Our minds actually send us messages

> **SINCE "DIETING" AND "WORKING OUT"**
> are relatively new concepts for
> human beings, it is as if we are
> going against our own instincts.

that give us long lists of really good reasons to stop
dieting and exercising. Our minds may be hardwired
to say yes to food and no to exercise.

This is why self-talk is important. When it is time
for a workout, our minds will begin to go through a
list of possible reasons that allow us to skip that
workout. Almost everyone's mind works in this way.
Call them "excuses" because that is the purpose they
serve. With food, we will search for a good reason to
consume the foods we know are not on our diets.
Have you ever said to yourself, "Well, it is a special
occasion. I'll just have a *little* bit of the cake." Or with
exercise, one might say, "It is cold outside. I can't

work out in the cold." Then tomorrow there is another reason. My experience with bariatric patients tells me that this internal dialogue of excuses will never go away.

Many times, the excuses may be true. The gym may be very expensive, and it may be very cold outside. That's not why they are excuses. They are called excuses because we don't find a way around them. We don't exercise inside if it is cold. We let the excuses stop us from exercising. Accept that excuse-making is normal, natural, and part of life. Your challenge as a bariatric patient is to learn to ignore the excuses by overriding them through positive self-talk and behavioral strategies. Those that successfully lose the weight and keep it off are the ones that learn to recognize the excuses and choose to ignore them.

THOSE THAT SUCCESSFULLY lose the weight and keep it off are the ones that learn to recognize the excuses and decide not to listen to them.

You will want to listen to them. Learning to override them is one of the most important keys to long-term success.

One of my patients calls this the "devil on my shoulder." He says "I know what I'm supposed to do, but I have the devil on my shoulder telling me why I really don't have to. It's a constant struggle." When it comes to diet and exercise, there is a vast difference between knowing what to do and actually doing it. Use the power of the mind to tip the scales in your favor. You can win over the devil on your shoulder. Let's consider two different scenarios:

1. Mary gets out of bed and has a shower. Afterward she looks in the mirror and says to herself, "You look disgusting. How could you ever go out in public looking like this?" Her self-talk will now influence how she feels. She will likely leave for work feeling down, self-conscious, negative about the day, and not motivated to eat properly or exercise. As her day progresses and lunch approaches, she may make poor choices, asking herself, "What difference does it make anyway?" In the afternoon she has a big piece of her coworker's birthday cake, rationalizing, "This will be my last piece. I'm really going to hit the diet hard tomorrow." When she gets home she does not exercise, deciding, "It's been a hard day. I'll do it tomorrow." This cycle perpetuates itself as she feels even worse the next day.

2. Mary gets out of bed and has a shower. Afterward she looks in the mirror and says to herself, "I am looking strong. I will take care of myself today, and tomorrow I will be even stronger and healthier. I'm a winner." Her self-talk will now influence how she feels. She will likely leave for work feeling better about herself and more motivated to eat properly and possibly exercise. When lunchtime approaches, she again uses positive self-talk by saying, "A healthy lunch will make me feel better, lose a little weight, and I'm worth it." She orders an appropriate lunch. Later, at the company birthday party, she says no thank-you to the cake because, "It's not worth the calories. I'd have to

walk three miles to walk that off." When she gets home, she is tired from a hard day, but says to herself, "I can manage 30 minutes of walking. I'll feel better than if I skip it." This cycle perpetuates itself as she feels better the next day.

✓ TO DO

Make your long-term goals part of your own self-talk. If your choice is between eating the treat or not eating the treat, you will probably end up eating it. But if your choice is between eating the treat and working toward good health and you say to yourself, "I am working toward a healthier life, and I already feel better," you will have a better chance of saying no to the treat.

Remember how it works:

- **Positive self-talk** creates positive feelings, which in turn lead to positive behavior.
- **Negative self-talk** creates negative feelings, which in turn leads to negative behavior.

Again, wanting to cheat on a diet is normal, but you can greatly increase your control over eating and exercise if your self-talk motivates you and increases your determination.

Example: Picture yourself at the grocery store. Listen to your self-talk that goes something like this: "I know I'm on a diet, but that doesn't mean my kids (or spouse) should be deprived of their favorite cookies." This is one of many excellent excuses for bringing inappropriate foods into the home and is of course the first step toward cheating. This type of self-talk allows

Tip

Our excuses may be very clever. If you find yourself
skipping workouts or eating the wrong foods, ask
yourself why. Is this an excuse? What am I really doing?
What are the consequences if I eat this or if I skip
exercise?

us to pre-plan our cheats by having these foods in the
house. It also sets up our environment for diet disaster.

We all know that being on a diet is no fun and
quickly becomes boring. We miss eating what we like,
and we look for excuses to break our diets. Remember
that sticking to the prescribed diet after surgery is
much like sticking to any other diet, and you will
encounter the same temptations, negative self-talk,
and excuse-making that you have in the past. Even
though these thoughts are normal, they will eventually
keep you from your weight loss goals unless you learn
to control them. Whatever thoughts came between you
and success in the past will likely occur again. The
best defense is to expect it and be ready with a
strategy.

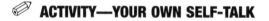 ## ACTIVITY—YOUR OWN SELF-TALK

1. **Spend several days tuning into your own
   self-talk.** Become aware of the rationalizations
   and justifications you give yourself to eat
   something that is not on your diet. Then decide
   you will not listen to this talk and that you intend
   to be successful.

2. **Make a list of positive phrases you can say to
   motivate yourself.** Every day will bring many

opportunities to cheat on your diet, and having a few positive and realistic lines to get you through will be key to your success.

Examples:

"Food is not my friend."

"I have power over food; it does not own me."

"I'm feeling better than I have in years."

3. **Use your new positive self-talk when in stressful eating situations.** Keep the phrases that work, and discard those that don't.

4. **Expect to experience heightened anxiety when choosing not to eat in these eating situations.** Remember that anxiety is only a feeling. It can't hurt you. It will go away. Use your self-talk, and if all else fails remove yourself from the situation completely. An escape route is always an option.

5. **If anxiety is a problem, use a deep breathing technique.** Take five slow, deep breaths, and remind yourself why you had bariatric surgery.

6. **Utilize the Thought-Stopping Technique.** This is a strategy for stopping a negative or self-defeating thought in its tracks. The second you realize you are having one of those thoughts, do two things:

   A. Picture a large, red stop sign in your mind.

   B. Say "STOP" to yourself.

   This will help you clear your mind so you may proceed with replacing the thought with one that will assist you in meeting your goals. An alternative to the stop sign is to wear a rubber band around your wrist and snap it gently when you find your thoughts are out of control. Either one will work until it becomes second nature for you.

CHANGING NEGATIVE SELF-TALK TO MORE REALISTIC TALK

At times, our negative self-talk becomes completely unrealistic. During these times, it is useful to know how to change that negative thought to a more realistic one. An example of negative or destructive self-talk would be, "I've had a terrible day. What would it hurt if I just had some of my old comfort foods for dinner? I'm miserable without my favorite foods. Maybe I shouldn't have had the surgery." Obviously the person in this example is on his way to cheating. He can avert diet disaster by listening to his own self-talk, recognizing how it makes him feel, and deciding to make changes. He may use a Thought-Stopping Technique, and then replace that negative thought with one more likely to benefit his health and help him meet his weight loss goals.

An example of more realistic and positive self-talk would be, "I'm progressing daily, I can walk two miles now, and I couldn't walk out the door three months ago. I'm feeling good, and that's all that matters. I can do this."

✓ TO DO

1. Tune into self-talk.
2. Recognize excuses.
3. Use the Thought-Stopping Technique (see page 50).
4. Override excuses.
5. Replace excuses with realistic self-talk.

MOTIVATIONAL VISUALS

A variation of self-talk is having a motivating picture that you can use to say "no" in familiar eating situations.

✓ TO DO

Use your mind as a photo album that shows the future. You will open that photo album in your mind when needed. The album should contain photos of yourself in your future. You are at your goal weight. What are you doing? What are you wearing? Who are you with? You are happy, healthy, and enjoying yourself.

Use your mental photo album any time. Your mental photo album provides a visual of the best aspects of your goals and will assist in keeping you on track.

Chapter 4

Stress Relief and Comfort Without Food

OBJECTIVES
1. List ways we learn habits and behaviors
2. List healthy ways to cope with stress without food

Food is the all-American stress reliever. We eat because we are hungry, and we eat for many other recreational and emotional reasons, such as boredom, stress, excitement, tradition, habit, depression, anger, comfort, and celebration. This behavior is normal in our society, and most of us were raised this way. Just about every social activity revolves around food in some way. Food is almost always the main event. From dating, to movies, to weddings, to holidays, food is a constant. The advertising industry spends billions of dollars per year to keep all of us eating for recreational or emotional reasons.

Even though it is normal, many people have gained large amounts of weight living this way and find it very difficult to alter their lifelong habits of eating because of these emotional/recreational habits. The surgery will likely decrease your perception of hunger, but it will not help to stop your recreational or emotional eating, since this type of eating is not based on hunger cues. The key to gaining control over emotional eating is all in the mind.

...YOU WILL FEEL A HEIGHTENED sense of anxiety when you cannot eat the foods you used to love or must stop after just a couple of bites.

Life after surgery will be stressful in ways you may not have considered. For example, what will you do on your first Thanksgiving, or your first dinner out at your favorite restaurant, or your first date? If you follow the tips provided in this book you will most likely do well, but you will feel a heightened sense of anxiety when you cannot eat the foods you used to love, or must stop after just a couple of bites. This anxiety is normal, but you must learn some healthy ways to cope with the emotions caused by drastically altering your lifestyle.

Stress affects all of us, and some more than others. Stress is an important factor to consider when deciding whether or not to have bariatric surgery. Most people greatly underestimate the difficulty involved in drastically changing a lifestyle. How many times have you vowed to change, only to slip back into old patterns within a few months? People who are not stressed often become that way after surgery. If you are already stressed, you may become overwhelmed. How you deal with stress will either improve your ability to adhere to lifestyle changes after surgery or make it more difficult for you to achieve your goals. Stress is an eating trigger for many people. It can also make it difficult to focus on the long-term goals. Stress can make you feel tired and sap your energy and motivation, making it difficult to stick to healthy habits.

DEFAULT SETTINGS

Our comfortable old eating habits are like DEFAULT SETTINGS. When under stress, we often revert to that default setting of eating. Our default settings are the habits we try hard to resist when on a diet. They are the habits we engage in between diets. It requires focus to maintain a healthy diet and exercise routine when stressed. A crisis or big change in our lives redirects our focus, and we often begin to revert to our old habits. These default settings never really go away.

HOW ARE OUR ORIGINAL DEFAULT SETTINGS FORMED?

Our response to food and food-related cues is established over many years and in several different ways. First, as children we may have eaten when we were upset and food calmed us down. Or we were given a bottle when we cried and then we felt better. These connections can be by chance or by design. Eventually we learned to eat in certain situations because we knew we would feel better afterward. This is a type of conditioning that strengthens over time and with repetition.

A second way we learn is by associating a food with an unrelated, separate thing, such as beer with watching football, or having donuts on Friday mornings at work, or having a danish while reading the newspaper. Over time, we feel compelled to do the two things together and feel anxiety if we do not.

Yet another way we learn is by listening to what our parents told us. We learned to "clean our plates," and we were being good children for doing it. We also learned by observing others. We learned that eating is a

DON'T EXPECT THE SURGERY to give you willpower during stressful times. It is extremely helpful to gain control over your eating before the surgery.

big part of celebration, family parties, a memorable Thanksgiving, and most other holidays.

These experiences form the basis of our default settings. They represent our early learning and connections that have been strengthened over many years of repetition. Breaking these connections is difficult because they are often connected to feelings of safety, security, celebration, family, and other intense emotions.

To break these habits, we must repeatedly break the connection between the newspaper and the danish and eventually the compulsion to eat while reading the newspaper will diminish. At the same time, a bariatric patient may begin to establish new default settings by drinking a protein shake while reading the paper.

- It is possible to set new defaults, but it takes time and conscious effort. In times of personal crisis or stress, we have a tendency to revert to the old settings. This is when it becomes important to pay special attention to our habits of eating and exercise so we will resist reverting to old habits.

- Excuses are our subconscious way of allowing us to slip back to our default settings. Learn to recognize these and say NO.

In emotional situations, there can be additional stress on bariatric patients because of the conflict between wanting to eat for comfort and not wanting to cheat. Most people do not realize how stressful this is, and many people do cheat.

Don't expect the surgery to give you willpower during stressful times. It is extremely helpful to gain control over your eating before the surgery. If you already had the surgery and are now finding yourself eating for emotional reasons, it is time to work on the problem using the techniques listed here. The surgery only keeps you from being hungry for a few months. It does nothing to stop emotional food cravings.

I ask people how they deal with stress, and almost everyone lists several healthy coping strategies. Most people also list eating as a favorite stress reducer after a hard day. Before surgery, or just after surgery, it is very important to have a few healthy coping strategies, or you may find yourself resorting to food for comfort. If you must eat to cope with stress, make sure it is something allowed on your diet.

HEALTHY WAYS TO DEAL WITH STRESS AND ANXIETY

Aim to utilize a few of these great stress relievers during your week.

1. Talk to a friend or family member about your feelings.
2. Spend time in a social activity not related to food.
3. Go to a movie, play, concert, or sporting event.
4. Take a leisurely drive and listen to music.
5. Go to the library, mall, or bookstore.
6. Go to the park with the dog, the kids, a friend, or alone.
7. Meditate.
8. Use Progressive Muscle Relaxation tapes (see sample script on page 59).
9. Exercise.
10. Do some stretching.
11. Write down your thoughts in a journal or diary.
12. Use the computer.
13. Get involved in a hobby or craft.
14. Reward yourself for all your hard work with something new.
15. Plan a vacation.
16. Get involved in a home improvement project.
17. Do some volunteer work.
18. Doodle, draw, or paint.
19. Learn a new skill, such as a sport or a language.
20. Make a list of all the things you will do when you achieve your weight goal.
21. Listen to relaxing music.
22. Use positive and motivating self-talk—give yourself a pep talk.
23. Take a hot bath.
24. Do some research on your home town and do some "tourist" activities.

25. Practice deep breathing exercises.
26. Close your eyes for a few minutes and visualize a safe, relaxing place.
27. Schedule time for yourself so you don't feel rushed.
28. Simplify your life whenever and wherever possible.

There is really no end to the possibilities. Any activity that calms you down or takes your mind off your stressors is a good choice. Whatever you do instead of eating will likely be a distant second to eating. Food has worked in the past and provided that comfort or calming effect. It may take months or even years to replace food with an acceptable alternative. A realistic expectation is that your alternative activity or relaxation technique will get your through the moment, but it will not work as well as food for some time. If you can overcome the crutch of food dependency, you will succeed.

Progressive Muscle Relaxation (PMR)

PMR is based on the fact that it is impossible to be stressed out and relaxed at the same time. Relaxation is the antidote to stress. Most of us know what it is to feel stressed and less stressed but seldom truly relaxed. PMR teaches you what complete relaxation really feels like. If you practice this several times per week for several weeks, you will be able to relax faster and will feel less stressed in situations that may cause stress for you now. Since stress is a powerful eating trigger for many people, think of PMR as a defense against emotional eating.

PMR teaches you to alternatively tense and then relax each muscle group in your body. By doing so, you will learn to relax more deeply than usual. This is helpful during the holidays, a personal crisis, or major changes in your life.

Instructions: Read the following very slowly into a tape. Pause for 3 to 5 seconds between each phrase where you see dots. Then play the tape several times per week when you can find about 12 minutes to be alone. Sit in a comfortable chair in a place relatively free of distractions.

[START OF TAPE]

Just lean back in your chair. Make yourself comfortable. Place both feet flat on the floor. Rest your hands comfortably in your lap. You may hear noises, but they will not influence your experience.

Begin by stretching your legs as far as they can go…Relax…Stretch your legs again… Point your feet up, toward you… hold…turn your feet down, away from you…hold…relax.

Now, tighten the muscles in your calves and in your thighs…tight…hold it…hold it….relax…

Feel the difference…

Let your legs go back, slowly, down to their original position…and relax all the muscles in your feet…all the muscles in your calves…and the muscles in your thighs…let your legs be completely relaxed…and now feel that wonderful relaxation coming up from your toes…up your calves…and your thighs…feeling nicely relaxed…very calm…and…very relaxed…calm and relaxed…just focus on your legs and feel your relaxation…

Now, stretch out your arms…make two fists…tighten the muscles in your fingers…feel the tightness…hold it, hold it…and relax…let your arms go down to their resting position…feel that relaxation…now stretch your arms again…tighten the muscles in your wrists, in your lower arms, in your upper arms…hold it, hold it…and, let go, just let go, let your arms go down to their original position…stop for a second, and take your time to notice that quieting feeling of relaxation through your fingers…through your hands…through your lower arms, and upper arms...let your arms go completely limp...take your time to increase that feeling of relaxation...very warm...very relaxed... calm... relaxed and calm.

Now, tighten the muscles in your back...now your chest...your abdomen...and your neck...hold it...hold it...let go of the tension. Just let go of the tension... Notice your muscles relax...take time to feel the muscles relax in your chest...in your abdomen...in your neck...all over your back...all your muscles feel nicely relaxed...

Now tighten the muscles in your face, first the muscles around your forehead, then the muscles around your eyes...make them tighter...hold it...hold it...now relax...tighten the muscles of your cheeks...the muscles around your mouth...the muscles of your chin. Make them tighter...hold it...and relax. Let all the muscles in your face relax, first the muscles of your cheeks, the muscles around your eyes, the muscles of your forehead...let all the tension drain from your face...let you chin sag if that feels good...take your time to enjoy the feeling of relaxation...very relaxed...and very calm...relaxed and calm...

Now breathe in through your nose, slowly and deeply, and hold it...hold it...and slowly breathe out through your nose....feel the relaxation...breathe in...breathe out...relax...

Once again take a very deep breath, hold it...hold it...and slowly let it out...let go of all your tension...your frustrations...your anxieties...feeling more and more relaxed...relaxed and calm...

Now take some time to scan your body...if you notice any tense spot...take your time to release that tension...very good...very relaxed...relaxed and calm...

Now, take time to breathe in and out...slowly begin to stretch your body...when you feel ready...slowly open your eyes...and focus on your surroundings...you will be ready to continue your day...relaxed and calm...focused and attentive...[END TAPE]

Chapter 5

The 3-Point Plan

OBJECTIVES

1. Describe the 3-point plan
2. List steps for successfully attending a party while adhering to the bariatric diet
3. List steps to going out to a restaurant after bariatric surgery while still enjoying yourself
4. State the reason why snacking is associated with weight regain after surgery
5. Describe steps to approaching the holidays that will assist in weight loss goals

You can inoculate yourself for stressful situations full of conflict and emotions and give yourself a better chance of success by following this strategy. Before you go into any situation that is likely to be difficult or in which you previously ate whatever you wanted, devise a plan. Think about three things that make up our 3-point plan:

A. What you will say to yourself
B. What you will say to others
C. What you will do.

Rehearse your plan mentally several times and when you go to the event you will be much less likely to do something regretful. This strategy has worked for many people I have counseled, and it can work for you.

Let's consider a hypothetical family gathering for which you need to devise your 3-point plan (what you say to yourself, what you say to others, and what you will do). How will you get through the evening without eating too much or eating the wrong foods?

A. WHAT YOU SAY TO YOURSELF

Some people say to themselves, "This is about my health, and I'm a healthy and different person now." Some say, "Food got me into this situation, and I'm not going to let it beat me." Or "This is about my family, not the food." Or "I'm worth it." With practice, you will find the phrases that get you through the tough spots. I advise everyone to begin experimentation before surgery with self-talk, and start a list of phrases that work for you. Say your motivating phrases when you feel like cheating or when you feel anxiety because you are not eating something you want.

Now that you have a couple of phrases of positive self-talk to help during your family gathering, the next step is to think of what to say to other people.

B. WHAT YOU SAY TO OTHERS

Some people like to be open in conversation about the surgery, and others feel it is a private matter. The most important thing is to be aware of how you are most comfortable and plan your strategy with that in mind.

When Uncle Charlie pressures you to try his famous potato salad, you will need to be prepared with a response. Perhaps you can say, "That sure looks good. Will you make it for me again in six months when I can try a bite?" The key is not to give in to pressure and to have a response that allows you to stay in control. Some patients tell me they eat all the wrong foods at gatherings because they do not wish to alienate anyone.

C. WHAT YOU WILL DO

The third part of the strategy is to plan what you will do when in the situation. This step involves the behavioral logistics of the party. For example, you may plan to avoid the hors d'oeuvres table, keep a glass of water in your hand, and have any conversations far away from the food. When the dinner arrives, you may plan to have three bites of the meat and two of the vegetable, and leave the table if it becomes overwhelming for you. The possibilities are endless, but the point is to have a workable plan prior to the party, and it should be a comfortable strategy.

> *Hint*
>
> Savor your food and enjoy it. It is really only a matter of quantity. This way you will feel less deprived.

D. MENTAL REHEARSAL

Whatever your plan is, it is helpful to rehearse mentally before you arrive. This will help you stick to it. Some basic tips to mental rehearsal are to sit in a quiet place and picture the scene in your mind. Be sure to use all your senses with this technique. The more vivid the scene, the better. Think of what you will hear, smell, see, taste, and how the air will feel over your skin. You will most likely experience an increased sense of control and find your experience unfolds closer to your ideal plan than if you had not used mental rehearsal. This is a popular technique with professional athletes because it works.

Even if mental rehearsal is not used, be sure to think about what you will say to yourself, what you plan to do, and what you will say to others prior to arrival.

Planning ahead in this manner offers a much better chance of success than simply hoping for the best or relying on others to keep you from eating. This proactive planning will put you in control and boost your confidence as well.

Now you can apply your 3-point plan to various situations you will experience as a bariatric patient. Let's take a look at several of these situations.

YOU'VE BEEN INVITED TO A PARTY

Going to a party for the first time after surgery can be both exciting and overwhelming. This may be the first chance for your friends to see you after having lost a couple of sizes. Remember to have your 3-point plan prepared and mentally rehearsed prior to arrival at the party—what you will say to yourself, what you will say to others, and what you will do. For many, this is the first real test after surgery, and it can be highly anticipated, dreaded, or something in between.

Your weight loss will likely be the subject of much conversation. You have reason to be proud, but not everyone is comfortable being the center of attention. You have worked hard and gone through many changes in order to be where you are. If possible, enjoy the attention.

Tips

1. Once during the evening, go to the hors d'oeuvres table. Take a few items and nibble. Don't worry about throwing some away if you take too much. If this is difficult for you, consider eating before the party and commit to just talking and sipping your drink. For some, it may be easier to avoid the food altogether than to eat a preplanned amount.

2. Keep a glass of water, iced tea, or other flavored water or non-caloric drink in your hand for sipping throughout the party.

3. Try to steer your conversations away from food. Remember to concentrate on the activity rather than the food.

4. You can discuss your weight loss or not, but the choice is yours. It is acceptable to ask that the subject be changed if you wish. On the other hand, it may be motivating for you to discuss it with people. It is entirely up to you.

5. Have a plan for how you will leave the party if you begin to feel overwhelmed. Always have an escape route. Some plan ahead to spend only two hours.

It is normal to feel as though others are watching you as you eat at the party. They are probably curious as to what you are able to eat. You may enjoy the attention, or you may feel uncomfortable. Plan your strategy with the idea that people will be curious. On the other hand, chances are they are not paying quite as much attention as you think they are.

Try to relax by using some of your relaxation techniques, such as deep-breathing or calming self-talk, if anxiety is a problem for you. If you prepared yourself properly, you will begin to feel comfortable in a short period of time.

When you leave, having followed your plan, pat yourself on the back. It is not easy going into a situation where you previously may have consumed food and/or alcohol. You are on your way!

YOUR FIRST DINNER OUT IN A RESTAURANT

This is a big test for the bariatric patient who has recently had surgery. Your first decision will be what to say to the waiter. Some people like to mention they have just had surgery and will need their food prepared according to specific guidelines. Others are a bit more private and would rather just order their food without butter or oil and with sauces on the side. Either way, you can order from the appetizer menu and most likely be full, or you can order from the dinner menu, eat your regular portion, and take the rest home.

Some of my patients like to split dinners in restaurants. You will find the method that suits you with time, but it is your choice whether or not to disclose that you have had surgery. It is not necessary to tell a waiter why you order a particular way, unless it makes you feel more comfortable.

A common fear is, "What if the food gets stuck or I have a problem at the restaurant?" The first bite often determines how the rest of the meal will be tolerated. Be sure to take your time and chew your food thoroughly. Anxiety about eating in a restaurant can make it difficult to swallow, so remember to relax and take slow deep breaths if you're feeling anxious. You may also request a table near the restroom. The host will probably be grateful for a chance to seat someone there voluntarily. If the worst does happen, it is not the end of the world. Simply get up from the table and walk to the restroom. Chances are you will be fine. Welcome back to the world of restaurants.

Tips

1. Choose a restaurant where you can order your meal prepared to your specifications. You may ask for your food without butter or oil or with sauces and dressings on the side.

2. Keep your mind on the activity of socializing rather than on the food itself.

3. Have your 3-point plan prepared and mentally rehearsed.

4. Ask to take the leftovers home with you, or better yet, ask for a "to-go" container as soon as your food arrives. Place most of the meal in the container before you begin eating. This strategy also assists with the "clean plate" compulsion. In this way you can be a member of the clean plate club without overeating.

5. Concentrate on the people you are with and the interesting conversation rather than just the food itself.

6. Begin to notice the sounds, sights, and smells in the restaurant. Take it all in. There is so much more to the experience than just the food.

7. Enjoy the food, too! The only difference is quantity. Savor it and enjoy it.

8. Some restaurants will allow bariatric patients to order from the children's menu, but be careful what you get. These meals are often high in fat.

THE HOLIDAYS ARE HERE!

It starts on Thanksgiving and ends on January 1. This is the time of year when we traditionally let go and enjoy large amounts of food without worrying about calories. It is a part of our upbringing and culture. Everyone else is doing it, and we do not want to feel deprived. Along with all the cheer and gift giving is food—and lots of it. How do you keep from gaining weight or significantly slowing down your weight loss during this time period? By planning.

Realize it is human nature to let down your guard during the holidays. The psychological connections are so strong, it is difficult to maintain healthy habits, but not impossible. I always find an influx of patients coming to support groups in mid-January. The usual complaint is they fell off the wagon in November and have been eating much more than recommended through the New Year. Many have gained weight and stopped exercising. Planning is the key to surviving the holidays with minimal disruption in your bariatric diet and exercise plan. It is possible to maintain your weight or even lose a bit.

✓ TO DO

1. **Just after Halloween, sit down and really think about the holidays.** Ask yourself what are the foods you are most interested in during this time and what are the foods you would be willing to give up for health. Make a list of foods you choose to keep. These are usually the ones that have the most meaning or are your favorites. Also list the ones you are willing to give up. These are usually the filler foods or snacks that are present during the holidays but that you could live without. Keep the lists handy, as you will need them when Thanksgiving approaches.

2. **Next, set up some rules while you have a level head unclouded by holiday excitement.** An example might be to allow yourself an alcoholic beverage once per week and choose the specific day. Another example might be to try your

Problem

"My pouch is bigger, and I can eat more, so I am overeating."

Solution

Shift your thoughts from "I must eat until I am full," to "I must eat only until I am no longer hungry." Remember it is not necessary to fill the pouch to capacity.

mother's sweet potato casserole, but only three or four bites on the holiday itself. The idea is to have what you really love, without adding all the other mindless calories. You can do this and still maintain your dietary regimen.

3. **Commit to following your diet as though it were not the holidays with the exception of the special foods on your holiday list.**

4. **Commit to continuing and even increasing your exercise regimen during the holidays.** Many are tempted to stop during this period, but exercise can limit the damage done by the extra food. Life gets more hectic during the holidays, but there is always time for exercise. Remember the benefits of added energy and stress reduction that exercise provides. It is very difficult to restart an exercise program once you let it go. Exercise should remain constant throughout the holidays.

5. **Ask your family for assistance.** Share the lists with them and ask that they not bring these foods to your home.

6. **Consider having holiday meals at another person's home instead of having the family to your house that first year.** Don't put yourself in too many situations where willpower dictates your choices and your health.

If all else fails, go to the section of this book called Emergency First Aid. I often get frantic phone calls from patients who cannot seem to get back on track. With preplanning and sensible rules, you will do well during this time of year.

YOU CAN STILL COOK FOR THE FAMILY WHILE ON THIS DIET

Another situation that will need preplanning is how to cook for the family and for yourself. It is always a good idea to discuss this with your family prior to surgery so everyone will know what to expect. There is no universal way to handle this, and it will depend on the dynamics of your family and what you are able to handle.

One of the easiest ways to prepare dinner for everyone is to prepare a protein, such as fish or hamburger. It can be prepared in many healthy ways, and you simply eat less than everyone else. Include a vegetable and other side dish for the family, and you are ready. This method allows you to eat the same foods as the rest of your family. It is healthy for the

Tip

Begin to think in terms of quality versus quantity. You will be able to eat many of your favorite foods eventually, but in much smaller amounts. You are not deprived, just eating smaller quantities.

family and is easier on you because you will not have to resist some forbidden food they may be having. It is important for some people to not feel like an outsider at mealtimes because that may be a stimulus for cheating.

On the other hand, a few people have told me they prefer having separate meals because it emphasizes that they are on a very special program. If you fall into this category, you may decide to cook completely separate meals for the rest of your family. If you follow this course, do not be tempted to eat the food you're cooking for others. You may only be able to do this after several months on the diet and after developing a certain indifference to food and confidence in your self control.

WHEN YOU ARE NOT THE COOK IN THE HOUSE

What happens when you are expected to eat what someone else is cooking for you? You may decide that you will cook for yourself or may discuss with the family the idea of everyone eating healthier. The important point is that you don't put someone else in charge of your adherence to the diet. If the only way you can have the required foods is to cook them yourself, this may be your best bet. Another option is to find a local restaurant that will prepare food to your specifications.

CAN FUN FOODS BE A PART OF THIS DIET?

YES, absolutely. After an initial period on a liquid diet, and a step-up to pureed foods for a short time, you will be able to eat solid foods. Your program's dietitian or your surgeon will provide you with a list of things you are allowed to eat. While sticking to the diet you will lose weight, but there are countless exciting ways to cook the proteins that comprise the main portion of your daily food intake. I have seen dips, skewered and grilled chicken, and hors d'oeuvres that look delicious. Be creative. Just because you are on a restricted diet does not mean it has to be boring and repetitive. Also, keep your eyes open also for new cookbooks for bariatric patients.

> **I HAVE SEEN DIPS,** skewered and grilled chicken, and hors d'oeuvres that look delicious. Be creative. Just because you are on a restricted diet does not mean it has to be boring and repetitive.

TEENAGERS ON THIS DIET

If you are a teenager, it will be tempting to have your parents cook and shop for you. Consider the idea that it should not be your parent's responsibility. A much better idea is to plan for yourself by putting the items you need on the family shopping list. Food preparation after surgery is a very time-consuming activity, and this is YOUR lifestyle change. It involves planning ahead, shopping, cooking, cutting foods into small pieces, packing lunches, and can take many hours per week. You have been found to be mature and responsible if you have been cleared for this surgery, so this is an opportunity to really take charge of your own health.

Since you will eventually move out of the house and have to do it yourself, it makes sense to take responsibility from the beginning. Think of it as a part-time job that will require much preplanning, preparation, and energy. I advise all of my patients to take personal responsibility for their own lifestyle changes, especially teenagers. This way when you do move out of the house, it will be a much easier transition.

SNACKING

Snacking has been associated with regaining weight after surgery. It is possible to fill up the tiny pouch many more times during the day than your dietitian will recommend. Even though snacking is considered healthy for some before surgery, afterward it can cause problems. Be sure to eat only the snacks recommended by your dietitian. Some patients report snacking up to 15 times per day. This will translate into less weight loss overall and possible regain of weight down the line.

Chapter 6

Beginning a Consistent Exercise Program

OBJECTIVES

1. Identify why lifelong exercise is key to keeping weight off after bariatric surgery
2. Describe how self-talk influences motivation to exercise
3. Describe how to choose the type of exercise that is right for you
4. Describe how to start and keep an exercise log
5. List motivational tips for exercise
6. Describe the 5-Minute Rule
7. Create long-term and short-term exercise goals
8. Choose exercise rewards

There are many psychological tips and strategies to exercise adherence. When working with bariatric clients, I encourage them to start their exercise program well before having the surgery. Getting into the exercise habit prior to surgery increases your confidence and sets the stage for success.

Exercise is a very important component to a patient's life after bariatric surgery. Exercise during weight loss will help you stay more toned, feel more energetic, and become stronger. It can burn more calories and assist in the weight loss itself. But the real surprise to many people is that exercise is even more important after you reach your goal weight. Successful weight maintenance is a product of proper eating and continued exercise.

I have heard horror stories of people gaining weight back, either because they reverted to previous eating habits or because they did not continue to exercise. When I see someone for the pre-surgery psychological evaluation, I always discuss the importance of lifelong adherence to an exercise program.

Start by setting aside some time, at least five days per week, and get in the habit of exercising on those days. It is fine to just walk for 5 to 10 minutes if that is all you can manage at this time, or to stretch and use upper body weights for a few minutes. The most important aspect of preparation is to get into the habit of scheduled exercise and to overcome the excuses used to skip workouts. Consistency is the key. With time you will be able to walk farther or work out for longer periods of time. To succeed, you must get into the habit of exercising no matter what else is going on in your life.

I often hear people say, "I lost the weight and never exercised." It is possible to do that because the decreased food intake causes most of the weight to come off. However, it is very difficult to KEEP the weight off without exercise. People who choose this course are at a very high risk of being unsuccessful in the long run.

If you need another motivation to exercise, try this: Exercise is one of the best proven stress

Tip

Would you describe yourself as a stubborn person? I have found that self-labeled stubborn people do well after surgery if they take a couple of steps:

1. Tell others not to push you or to remind you of what you should be doing. Stubborn people have a tendency to do the opposite.

2. Tell yourself that you will not let anyone or anything get in the way of your goal. Tell yourself that nothing will keep you from exercise, and no one will convince you to eat something you should not. Tap into that stubbornness and use it to your advantage.

reducers, and new research shows that exercise can work about as well as an antidepressant—without the side effects. Also, since stress and depression are potent triggers to eat for many people, you can see how exercise can become a very important and powerful tool for weight loss and maintenance.

Exercise is for life—This is a harsh reality, but a fact of life nonetheless. Everyone knows someone who is thin, eats whatever he wants to eat, and never gains weight. It is unfair, but you are likely on the other end of the spectrum. Once you realize that it isn't fair, but it is reality, you are in a position to begin making lasting changes. For whatever reason, once a person gains weight, then loses weight, exercise is required to keep it off for life.

You may be exercising now. If so, you are way ahead of the game. You may have tried to start exercise programs numerous times but have been unable to stick with it, or perhaps you have never really exercised. Whatever your situation, this section will give you tips and techniques to get you going and keep you on track.

EXERCISE AND SELF-TALK

We all enjoy exercise immediately AFTER the workout. The problem occurs just before the workout when we start making excuses not to do it. How many times have you skipped a workout after saying to yourself, "I'm too tired," or "It's too late," or "It looks like it's going to rain," or "I don't have to exercise on vacation." The list of possible excuses is endless. This self-talk allows us to skip the workout, but deep down inside we know the truth. The next day we are feeling a bit sluggish and start with the excuses again. Often we end up saying, "I'll just start again tomorrow. I'll really get into it again tomorrow." Of course, tomorrow never comes.

Thoughts such as these are absolutely normal. Everyone, including surgeons, athletes, psychologists, and dietitians, battles these excuses daily. If you want to be successful with exercise maintenance, it is time to learn to ignore and override these excuses. It is not possible to stop exercising and keep all the weight off for life.

Consider the people who go on regular diet and exercise plans and lose substantial amounts of weight. Then they stop both exercise and healthy eating when they reach their goal. The weight returns, but they complain that the diet did not work. Actually the diet did work, but they did not make permanent lifestyle changes, rather they made the changes only until they reached the goal. If these people had simply continued to exercise, they would have likely kept most of the weight off. This type of thinking illustrates normal human responses to lifestyle changes. We tend to drift back into our old habits. It is exactly the same after bariatric surgery. Use your motivational techniques to avoid this trap. When you get to the maintenance stage, focus on your program, your habits, and avoidance of those excuses.

In order to motivate yourself, it helps to discover your long range goals. These goals will become part of your positive self-talk, and that will help motivate you to exercise even when you do not feel like it. Here are some tips to finding your internal motivation:

1. Perhaps you are experiencing a deterioration in health. Say to yourself one of the following: "I will exercise today because my health is the most important concern in my life right now;" "I can't wait to feel good again;" or "If I exercise today, I am one step closer to my goal of good health and feeling good again."

What are my excuses?

To find your own excuses, make a list of all the reasons you do not exercise, have skipped a workout in the past, or have ever quit an exercise program. Now look for ways around those reasons. For example, if you are exhausted after work, then try working out early in the morning. If the gym is closed when you want to work out, then buy some home equipment or just do some walking in your neighborhood. It is normal to have reasons not to exercise, but do not let those excuses keep you from your goal of losing weight and keeping it off for life.

2. If your real motivation is to look good, then say: "Each time I exercise, I get closer to my goal of looking great and wearing that bathing suit." You may wish to look at a picture of yourself when you were once at the weight you now hope to achieve, or use a magazine picture of your fantasy goal.

3. If your goal is to have energy to get involved in activities, then say, "A little work today will help me be able to hike in the woods with energy, or swim in the ocean, or shop at the mall without shortness of breath."

4. If your goal is to be able to keep up with the kids, then say, "I'm doing this for the kids. They are worth it, and they will love having an active parent again."

5. If your goal is to turn back the clock in general, then perhaps try, "I can't wait to feel good again, and exercise will get me there." Or "My spouse isn't going to recognize the new me."

Your motivation might include several of the above, or something else completely individual to you.

It is not uncommon for a patient to tell me that he or she just does not like exercise. He or she is often under the mistaken belief that everyone who exercises likes it. Sure, some people love exercise, but the vast majority do it because of the benefits. It is similar to brushing your teeth or taking a shower. When we are very young, we are taught these habits. Most of us resisted them. We might have pretended to take a shower or just dampened our towel or toothbrush. Eventually, we came to appreciate the benefits of tooth brushing and bathing. Now we would not dream of skipping our shower or not brushing our teeth. We don't do it because we enjoy it; we do it because we have to in order to be clean. I know of no one who looks forward to brushing their teeth.

> **ADDING ANY HABIT TO YOUR LIFE** is difficult, but one requiring time and effort, such as exercise, will take many years to become automatic, like brushing your teeth.

We learned these skills as children, and we do not question them now. Exercise will eventually become like that, but it will take years to get there. Can you imagine someone saying, "I'm just not a tooth brushing kind of person," or "I used to be a tooth brusher, but it was boring, and I was changing jobs so I was really busy and didn't have time to brush," or "My arm was sore so I stopped." The excuses may be true, but we would never let that stop us from brushing our teeth.

These excuses seem ridiculous when applied to brushing our teeth, but are routinely used to avoid exercise. Adding any habit to your life is difficult, but one requiring time and effort, such as exercise, will take many years to become automatic like brushing your teeth. Our minds actually work against us by providing a list of excuses so we do not have to exercise. Learn to recognize and override those excuses. Millions of people exercise every day, not because they like it and not because they are motivated but for one reason—to keep weight off.

STARTING THE EXERCISE PROGRAM

Starting an exercise program can be both exciting and frustrating. It takes approximately six months for exercise to become a habit. Some people will learn to love exercise and some never will. For the first few weeks you will be more tired than usual, but if you stick with it, you will notice an increase in energy. Before long you will feel stronger and sleep better. Exercise is a natural antidepressant and is good for your heart. It is a stress reducer, decreases anger and hostility, and gives you a sense of control over your life. It may be one of the greatest things you can do for yourself, but it takes work.

EXERCISE is a natural antidepressant and is good for your heart. It is a stress reducer, decreases anger and hostility, and gives you a sense of control over your life. It may be one of the greatest things you can do for yourself, but it takes work.

One of the most elusive aspects of exercise adherence is making it a priority. As a bariatric patient, your health has to be the priority, and exercise is an integral part of your health. It may feel awkward asking your spouse to watch the kids so you can go walking or postponing making dinner so you can go to the gym, but it is necessary. Keep in mind that your insurance company, surgeon, and hospital staff are all on your team and working toward your good health. They are your cheerleaders and are there to help if you need it.

The idea of putting yourself first may be foreign and uncomfortable and may be followed by guilt, especially if you have always been the caretaker of the family. Push yourself through those feelings, and they will diminish with time. Remember that if you take care of yourself, you will be better able to take care of your family.

I have talked to many people who were able to change their eating habits, but who never became consistent with exercise. They did not think it was necessary because they were losing weight. Eventually they began to gain weight back. Exercise is one of the most important components to long-term weight loss maintenance. There is no way around that fact. It is not fair, but it is reality. Once you understand the necessity of adding exercise, you are halfway there.

HOW MUCH SHOULD I EXERCISE?

The professionals in your bariatric surgery program will likely vary on this answer. Most will tell you to gradually increase to 3 to 5 times per week or more and for at least 30 to 45 minutes per workout. If you can make it part of your daily routine, that is even better. Aerobic exercise is excellent, and adding free weights or equipment is a good supplement. Walking is a great way to begin, and it is inexpensive, simple to do, can be done from home, and can be as easy or intense as you choose. Whatever your choice of exercise, remember to discuss it with your doctor.

Start small. If all you can do is walk for two minutes, then that is a good place to start. Perhaps by the next week you will be able to walk 3 or 4 minutes. Think of an exercise continuum where you are at one end (at the beginning) and Olympic athletes are at the other end. You may never be an Olympian, but at least now you are on that same continuum.

The most important part in the beginning is just getting into the habit of working out. It seems simple, but this is one of the most difficult phases of exercise. Battle that negative self-talk and ignore the excuses. Making these excuses is normal, and all people that exercise experience them, but they are what stands between you and your goal.

START SMALL. If all you can do is walk for two minutes, then that is a good place to start.

Here is a helpful strategy. If you skip a workout for any reason, say to yourself, "I choose not to exercise." This helps to keep the right perspective on exercise and assists in taking responsibility for skipping workouts rather than using some external factor as the reason. It is easy to blame skipping workouts on having "no time," but realistically there is time; we just choose to use it for something other than exercise. Make a commitment to yourself that if there is not enough time to exercise, something else will have to go, not the exercise. Perhaps the dog gets a bath tomorrow, or maybe the bills get paid later in the evening. There is always time for exercise if you make it a priority.

DO I HAVE TO SPEND A LOT OF MONEY TO JOIN A GYM?

You absolutely do not have to spend a lot of money by joining a gym. Going to the gym is not for everyone. You can exercise from your home and still achieve your weight loss and weight maintenance goals. On the other hand, some people enjoy the camaraderie, easy access to personal trainers, access to top-of-the-line equipment, and available support. It is an individual decision, and some have both a gym membership and a home exercise program.

WHAT EXERCISES SHOULD I CHOOSE?

Boredom is the enemy in an exercise program. Try activities you are interested in or ones that you may have enjoyed in your past. Choose between walking, rollerblading, swimming or pool walking, joining a gym, bicycling, hiking, water aerobics, tennis, golf without a cart, using free weights, mall walking, and many others. Some people choose several activities and alternate depending on their mood. Expect exercise to be boring most of the time, but you are not doing it for entertainment. You are doing it for your health and your future. On the other hand, some people really find they enjoy exercising and look forward to it. Others set goals and achieve amazing things they thought would never be possible. I have met people that have completed marathons and triathlons and climbed mountains. They found an inner athlete. Perhaps there is one in you.

ARE THERE ALTERNATIVES TO THE 30 to 40 MINUTE WORKOUT?

Sure. An interesting variation is to do three or four 10-minute workouts during the day. It may be easier to fit in 10 minutes on the treadmill four times than to set aside one larger block of time. To take this route requires extraordinary determination because you must motivate yourself to exercise several times each day. It is also helpful to purchase

AN INTERESTING VARIATION is to do three or four 10-minute workouts during the day. It may be easier to fit in 10 minutes on the treadmill four times than to set aside one larger block of time.

a pedometer to wear all day. By the time you reach your goal weight, you should be able to accumulate at least 10,000 steps per day.

Either way, you need to choose to exercise. Along with the long workout, or several short ones, you can also add small opportunities to burn calories throughout the day. Start parking farther away from your office building, grocery store, or mall. Take short energizing strolls throughout your workday. Walk the dog a bit farther than usual. It all adds up.

QUESTIONS

There are several other questions to ask yourself when making your exercise choice.

1. **How much will it cost to buy the equipment?** Be realistic about what is within your budget. You do not need to spend a lot of money or join a gym. Exercising from home is a good choice, and walking is inexpensive. All you need is a good pair of walking shoes.

2. **Will I have to travel to do the exercise?** Consider how accessible your choice will be. If you join a gym, there is an extra step to exercising as you must drive to the gym.

3. **Is there too much preparation time involved in doing my everyday workout?** Do you have to prepare a large amount of equipment? Is there a time commitment for maintenance of equipment?

4. **Is it something I think I will enjoy or have enjoyed in the past?**

5. **Do I need an exercise buddy to motivate me?** If you need a partner, then activities where you will be accountable for missing a workout would be a good choice for you. Perhaps joining a gym or having appointments with buddies or a personal trainer would be beneficial.

6. **Am I interested in this activity?** If it doesn't interest you, it will be next to impossible to sustain the exercise routine. Just because your friend likes water aerobics does not necessarily mean it will be a good choice for you.

7. **What will my backup exercise choice be if it is raining or my partner is unavailable?** Always have an exercise video, free weights, or some other type of physical activity planned for when nature interferes with Plan A.

8. **Will I actually do the exercise I choose or will I feel too self-conscious?** Be realistic. I have been told by many patients that they will not go to the gym until they have lost 50 pounds. If this describes you, then perhaps purchasing a stationary bicycle or doing exercises at home is a better choice on a temporary basis.

9. **If you have special needs or are not able to exercise due to pain or mobility, you will need to consult an exercise physiologist.** Most hospital programs have one on staff, and together you can creatively design an exercise program that will meet your needs. Some of my patients in wheelchairs do aerobic videos designed just for them. These videos emphasize upper body movements, and I have been told that they are enjoyable. As you lose weight and hopefully gain mobility, your exercise program will evolve.

KEEP AN EXERCISE LOG

An exercise log is a helpful tool for long-term success. It is motivating to see your progress and reinforcing to add another workout to the list. Another advantage to logging your workouts is the ability to look for trends. What time of day feels best to you for exercise? How many days per week of exercise works best for you? How does your workout feel if you missed a few days in a row? I know people who use their logs to track their feelings, their weight, and even major life events. Log books keep you honest. It motivates as well if you have to write "no workout" on skipped days.

Here is another trick. If you skip a workout you must write the reason in the log book. "No time" is not an option since there is always time to find at least 20 minutes. It may be at 5:00 am, or during lunch, or while catching the news in the evening, but in most circumstances there will be an opportunity to fit at least a short workout into your schedule. You must be very honest with yourself. If you have 30 minutes to watch TV, you have time to exercise. Challenge yourself to be as healthy as you have the potential to be.

In your logbook, you will indicate the activity you participated in, the time you spent doing it, and the speed or pace if appropriate. It is helpful to devise a rating system, such as a scale from 1 to 5, to rate your overall experience. When you achieve a 5, take

---

Exercise Log

Date:

Time:

Exercise:

Rating:

Comments:

_____

_____

_____

_____

_____

_____

Visit www.bariatrictimes.com for a downloadable PDF of this log.

Case Study

George had bypass surgery four years ago. At 410 pounds he had diabetes, high blood pressure, sleep apnea, and joint pain. He reached his lowest weight of 210 pounds about one year later. George was ecstatic. His diabetes and sleep apnea had disappeared, blood pressure was in the normal range, he took fewer medications, and his joint pain had significantly reduced.

He came to a group recently having regained over 80 pounds. He had been told by the surgeon to exercise, but he couldn't make himself do it. He would exercise once, and then stop for a week or two. He was aware of the repercussions of not exercising. He refused to go to therapy to work on the thoughts that keep him from exercising. He stated, "I just don't like exercise. I can't do it. I don't want to do it."

George disregarded his doctor's advice and never began to exercise. Without it, the prognosis is poor that he will ever lose the weight, and stop regaining. On his last visit, it was determined that his blood pressure was increasing and joint pain was returning.

note of the factors that contributed to such a great workout so you can recreate them.

There are several types of logs from which to choose. There are exercise logs available for purchase at most major book stores, and they come in many different sizes and price ranges. Some excellent software is also available for tracking workouts. The advantage to the software is the ease of entering data. All of your exercises, routes, and preferences can be entered beforehand, and keeping up with your log involves just a few keystrokes. If you are computer savvy, there are some free exercise logs on the Internet. You simply join a free site, are given a password, and can log your workouts online. With both the Internet and software, you can generate charts and graphs of your progress and most can track weight loss as well.

MOTIVATION TO EXERCISE

Let's face it. If motivating yourself to exercise was easy, we would all be out there daily. Motivation is inconsistent and often elusive. This section will address issues related to the difficulty most people experience in beginning and sustaining an exercise program.

When given the choice to exercise or not exercise, most people will choose not to exercise. Realistically, it is an effort. It's not much fun, and we would rather not do it at all. But that is not really the choice anymore. The real issue here is your health. Exercise is just a means to an end.

Motivation is not a trait. You are not naturally an unmotivated person. Chances are you are well motivated in many areas of your life. The challenge is to motivate yourself specifically for exercise.

Motivational tips. Since exercise motivation is a problem for most people, here are some tips that may help when you need it. Motivation can be high one week and low the next. Increasing motivation will likely be an issue for life. Listed are some motivational strategies for exercise. Experiment and see what works best for you.

1. **Play some upbeat music as you get dressed to exercise.**

2. **Buy some magazines that feature your sport or activity.** There are magazines for walking, running, bicycling, surfing, bodybuilding, hiking,

mountain biking, swimming, triathlon, and many others. Just seeing them sitting on your coffee table can help motivate you. You do not have to be a professional athlete to learn valuable information about your sport from these publications, and they can really get you excited about being involved.

3. **Join a group.** There are walking groups, swimming groups, groups that do only calisthenics, roller hockey teams, softball leagues, jazzercise, water aerobics clubs, and many others. The advantage of these is having other people counting on you to show up. If you know self-motivation is a problem, perhaps knowing others are expecting you will help. Playing on a team is a good idea if you enjoy the sport, and you would benefit from having an ongoing appointment for exercise.

4. **Along those same lines, it sometimes helps to make a pact with an exercise buddy.** Making a commitment to be there for your buddy can help you stay consistent with your program. However, if your exercise buddy cancels you must still exercise. The trap is that you may end up putting someone else in charge of your exercise program. Make a commitment that you will work out with your buddy, but if they are

Tip

Think of yourself as an athlete. If you are exercising at all, you are an athlete. You may be a beginner, but you are an athlete.

unavailable, you will still exercise. The buddy is the icing on the cake.

5. **Purchase a new piece of equipment or new workout clothes.**

6. **Enter an event, such as a three-mile walk for charity.** Listings are located on the Internet or in the newspaper. Get some others involved, and make it a group activity. Give yourself several months to work up to the distance.

7. **Set goals and rewards for sticking to your program** (Please refer to page 100 for more information).

8. **Increase the rhythm of your breathing slightly.** With each inhalation say the word "energy."

9. **Start a pre-exercise routine that gets you in the mood to exercise.** Olympic athletes use this technique. You might include stretching, repeating a motivating word to yourself, and listening to a favorite song as you dress for the workout.

10. **Use distractions, such as a portable radio, CD player, MP3 player, GPS speed/distance system, or talking pedometer.**

11. **Save an interesting mental activity for your workout, such as planning your wish list for the holidays, planning your next vacation, or planning your child's next birthday party.**

12. **Imagery is a powerful psychological technique.** It involves using your mind to create a vivid mental picture. Use energizing pictures like a locomotive or a tiger ready to pounce. These images will help you feel more energetic and ready to exercise. You may wish to imagine your body full of white energy. Whatever image is energizing to you is just right.

13. **While exercising, you can use imagery to help you through your workout.** For example, while walking or jogging you may imagine you are being pulled by a rope or pushed by a giant hand. Imagine you are in an exotic location or crossing a finish line in front of crowds of screaming fans. The possibilities are endless.

14. **Pay ahead.** If you want to eat something extra, don't say to yourself, "I'll exercise more tomorrow." Instead, pay ahead. Exercise more today, and then decide if you still want to eat that something extra.

15. **Use time management and organizational techniques and prioritize your schedule.** This will help to eliminate obstacles in your lifestyle change and give you more time for exercise.

16. **If you find yourself getting bored, change something.** Try a new exercise, vary your routine or route, or buy a new piece of equipment or clothing.

17. **Grandma's rule.** Remember when Grandma would tell you, "You can't have dessert until you eat your vegetables?" You probably did eat the brussel sprouts so you could have dessert. You can use this technique for exercise, too. Try, "I won't have dinner until I finish my three-mile walk," or "I won't surf the Internet until I go to the gym." The technique works.

18. **Hire a personal trainer.** Personal trainers are very motivating. Some even come to your house. Be sure to check their qualifications thoroughly.

THE 5-MINUTE RULE

There will be times when you find it almost impossible to motivate yourself to exercise. The 5-Minute Rule was designed to use in these "motivational emergencies." It is based on the reality that just getting started is the most difficult part.

CAN'T SEEM TO GET MOTIVATED? Tell yourself you only have to exercise for five minutes. Go ahead and put on your workout clothes and get started. If after five minutes you just can't go on for any reason...you may quit. At least you know you gave it the old college try.

Let's say you just can't motivate yourself today. Here's how the 5-Minute Rule works. Tell yourself you only have to exercise for five minutes. Go ahead and put on your workout clothes and get started. If after five minutes you just can't go on for any reason, even if it's just because you are not in the mood, you may quit. At least you know you gave it the old college try. You will probably feel more motivated the next day, rather than less motivated if you had completely skipped the workout. Sometimes magic happens. Most find that nine out of ten times you will choose to keep on exercising when your five minutes are up, because the hardest part is getting dressed and starting in the first place. Either way, you win. You end up doing the workout, or you feel like you at least tried.

GOAL SETTING

A little known and highly motivational technique is goal setting. Goals challenge you. They are extremely motivating, and it feels great when you achieve them. A goal or a series of goals is necessary to help direct your exercise, to keep you focused, and to keep you motivated.

There are two types of goals: long-term goals and short-term goals.

Long-term goals. These are the BIG goals. It may be to walk five miles, do a triathlon, play hockey, or ski for five hours straight. It is anything that may have seemed out of reach to you before.

Short-term goals. These are the STEPS needed to achieve the long-term goal. Often called "bite-sized goals," short-term goals should be:

1. *Realistic.* You may be able to only walk 100 yards at first. Do not set your sights too high. If you haven't

exercised in 20 years, give yourself a break. You can always add time, speed, or distance as you meet each short-term goal.

2. *Measurable.* You should be able to measure your progress in miles, time, number of days per week you work out, etc.

3. *Moderately difficult.* Research shows people work harder for goals that are not too hard and not too easy. Set the bar for yourself somewhere in the middle where you will be challenged but not too much.

4. *Specific.* Write out your goals. State how many days per week you intend to do what you have chosen. Depending on what activity you choose, you should also indicate the time you will take to do it, or the distance you will go. If you plan to walk two miles four times a week, you are likely to work harder to achieve that goal.

✓ TO DO

Write down your long-term goal and then the short-term goals you will use to achieve it. Plan your week each Sunday evening and attempt to adhere to your plan.

Example: My Goals and Plan

My long-term goal is to walk a 5K race (3.1 miles). I will choose a race that is five months from now.

1. My short-term goal is to walk 1/2 mile per day (about 10 to 15 minutes), four days per week for the first two weeks (Monday, Wednesday, Friday, and Saturday).

2. At Week 3, I will extend my walk to 3/4 of a mile (about 15 to 20 minutes), and by six weeks I will be walking one mile per day (about 20 to 30 minutes), four days per week.

3. At Week 8, I walk 1 to 1.5 miles per day (about 30 to 40 minutes), and two miles (about 40 to 50 minutes) by Week 10.

4. At Week 14, I will walk three miles (about 60 minutes) twice per week.

5. By Week 20, I will enter a 5K walk for charity.

REWARDS

Achieving goals is much more motivating if you attach a reward. If you can't motivate yourself for a health reason, how about a new DVD or new clothes?

There are two types of rewards: internal and external.

Internal rewards. These rewards are the physical and psychological benefits we get from doing the activity. They include a sense of accomplishment, pride, energy, strength, enjoyment, and feeling better. These are potentially present every time we exercise.

External rewards. These rewards are treats we promise ourselves for meeting our goal. It should be something you desire enough to work toward and something you would not ordinarily purchase for yourself. Some new clothes, a new CD, a mini-vacation, or a power tool are examples. Of course your pocketbook will dictate the types of rewards you plan, but the key is you only receive the reward if you achieve your goal. Another type of external reward is more intangible, such as a vacation day from work to use as you please. Whatever you choose, it can serve as a great motivator when you really need one.

You may choose a goal such as the Presidential Physical Fitness Award. It is available for adults, and information is on the Internet at www.fitness.gov. There are patches, certificates, and other motivational rewards for meeting requirements in 100

> **IT TAKES ABOUT SIX MONTHS** for exercise to become a habit. The external rewards will help get you to that point. After it becomes a habit, it will be more difficult to skip your workout, and the internal rewards may be enough to sustain your motivation.

different sports and activities, such as walking, bicycling, and aerobics. There is even a category for doing a combination of different activities.

It takes about six months for exercise to become a habit. The external rewards will help get you to that point. After it becomes a habit, it will be more difficult to skip your workout, and the internal rewards may be enough to sustain your motivation. You can reintroduce rewards into your program any time that you need them.

A large percentage of people quit their exercise programs. Do not let that be an option for you. Flip that switch in your mind from "I hope I have time to workout" to "Nothing will keep me from working out."

To be successful in sticking to your exercise program, remember these tips:

1. List your long-term and short-term goals, and attach rewards to your effort.
2. Log all workouts.
3. Use the motivational tips.
4. Prioritize exercise in your life. Your weight and health depend on it.
5. Do not expect instant results.
6. Give it a chance. It takes about six months to become a habit.
7. Learn to ignore that negative self-talk and turn it into positive self-talk.
8. Remember that exercise works to prevent weight regain in the maintenance stage of weight loss.

Chapter **7**

Behavior Modification

OBJECTIVES

1. Describe how our habits are formed
2. Create a seven-day food log
3. Analyze your food log for patterns in recreational and emotional eating
4. List behavior modification strategies for weight loss.

Most everyone has heard the term *behavior modification*, but few truly understand its application to diet and exercise. In this section, you will learn specific strategies to help you stay consistent and on track with your lifestyle change goals. These tips will greatly increase your ability to make these changes and help your transition to a healthier lifestyle.

Behavior modification is a set of small changes you can

make that will assist you in learning your new habits. Habits are very difficult to change, and certain aspects of your environment and some of your normal behaviors will make it even more difficult. Behavior modification is based on the idea that powerful psychological connections between certain cues and eating are established over time. Examples are watching football and eating chicken wings or coming home from work and immediately making a sandwich. These habits are normal for most of us but must be changed in order to be successful with weight loss. Because the psychological connections tend to be very strong, there is a tendency to fall back into old habits. These behavior modification techniques will make it easier to start new, healthier habits.

Habits in general are formed by repeating the action over time. New habits are formed in much the same way. Starting new habits is more difficult because it also involves resisting an old habit. This transition is stressful for most people. Refer to the section on stress reduction to help with this change. When we resist an old comfortable habit, we will usually feel some anxiety. This does not mean that you must go back to the old habit to feel better. A better alternative is to learn behavior modification techniques and cope with anxiety in a healthy way so you can progress with your lifestyle change goals.

When you attempt to change any habit, there will initially be anxiety. Learn to cope with the anxiety by using relaxation and deep breathing techniques. Power through the transition period and you will be successful at changing the habits that make weight loss difficult.

The first step to starting behavior modification is to figure out your particular triggers, cues, emotions, and situations that lead to emotional, recreational, or habitual eating.

✓ TO DO

All that is required for this activity is paper and a pen. For the next seven days, you will record everything you eat, what was going on at the time, and your emotions.

This activity can be completed before the surgery or after the surgery if you find yourself drifting back into old eating habits.

Spend one week recording everything you eat. Write down the time of day, what you ate, what was going on at the time, and the predominant emotion just before you ate (lonely, tired, stressed, happy, etc.). Write down everything, even if it seems insignificant. The payoff comes when you have a week or more worth of data to examine.

When you have at least seven days of information, sit down and look for patterns:

1. Are there one or more predominant emotions that seem to lead to eating?

2. Is there a particular time of day or night that appears to be more troublesome for you?

3. Is there a particular place that triggers eating?

4. Is there an activity that triggers eating, such as watching TV?

5. Is the presence of particular foods a trigger?

6. Is a particular day more of a problem than others?

7. What about automatic or mindless eating, such as snacking or nibbling while cooking?

8. Try to distinguish between internal cues (e.g., sadness, excitement) vs. external cues (e.g., television commercials or the scent of food cooking).

Once you have this information, you are in a much better position to begin making changes. When you understand the places, emotions, foods, time of day, and other patterns that lead you to eat, you can commit to avoiding these triggers, changing your environment or recreational pattern, and looking for alternatives. Change the routines that always lead to eating. The key is to become aware of the triggers, and then to make planned, alternative choices to avoid the trigger or change the situation.

As you begin to change these connections between cues and food, they will lose some of their power over you. They will always be there to some extent, but you will learn to take control of the situation rather than the situation control you.

SPECIFIC BEHAVIOR MODIFICATION STRATEGIES FOR WEIGHT LOSS

Begin to look at your home and work environment like a detective. What specific behaviors, habits, or aspects of your environment interfere with making lasting lifestyle changes? These cues can be eliminated or at least greatly diminished. Use the data you have from your food log to pinpoint the key problems and then try the following strategies:

1. **Eat only as advised by your bariatric doctor.**
Usually this will be three meals per day. Try not to
allow yourself to snack between recommended
meals while making this transition. If you must,
make it a bariatric-friendly snack.

2. **Eat very slowly and place your eating utensil
on the plate between bites.** As a bariatric
patient you will be advised to chew your food at
least 25 times, so this in itself will slow you down.

3. **Do not engage in other activity except
eating at mealtime.** Concentrate only on eating.
Avoid reading, watching television, or too much
conversation. This time is about eating only.

4. **It is most important to eat in a specific
place.** Choose a room where you will do all of
your eating, and promise yourself not to eat
anywhere else. If possible, eat in the same chair.
Do not eat while driving or doing other activities
as you will quickly lose track of the amount you
have consumed. It is important not to establish a
connection between driving and eating.

5. **Stay out of the kitchen except when
absolutely necessary.** Keep the kitchen light off
so the room is not so inviting, and try to take
alternate routes that don't lead you past it if
possible. Make sure food is stored only in your
kitchen.

6. **Use small plates, bowls, and utensils.**

7. **Do not keep leftovers on the table to invite additional nibbling after you finish.** Instead, get up from the table immediately and do something else. It may be helpful to store leftovers in the refrigerator before your meal so you will not be tempted to eat more later.

8. **Keep food out of sight as much as possible.** Do not keep it on the counter or in see-through containers. Keep your healthier choices in see-through containers so you learn to choose those before the others.

9. **Do not leave bowls of small snacking foods on the counter or table.** We will eat "one or two" every time we pass.

10. **Use these principles at work, too.** Take all snacks out of your drawers and off of your desk, including candy dishes for "clients or coworkers."

11. **Bring healthy snacks and meals with you to work so you will not be at the mercy of the cafeteria, fast food, or vending machines.**

12. **Do not eat lunch at your desk.** Go to the lunchroom or a picnic table outside, but break the psychological connection between your desk and eating.

13. **At break time, avoid the break room where others may be eating or where vending machines are located.** Instead, take a stroll outside or inside your building. Make phone calls, do some stretching, or balance your checkbook.

14. **Learn to change your routine.** If you go to the refrigerator first thing after work, learn to go directly to another room so you will eventually break that connection.

15. **Learn to read labels on grocery store items.** Shop only when you are not hungry, and bring a prepared list. Avoid certain aisles that might be tempting for you, like the crackers and cookies aisles, for example. There will be little or no food appropriate for a new bariatric patient in that aisle.

16. **Play soothing music while eating.** It tends to slow us down.

17. **Try not to nibble while preparing foods.** This is a common trap. We may not eat much at dinner, but we do not count all those bites taken during preparation. Plan ahead so you are not hungry while preparing meals, and try strategies such as brushing your teeth or keeping sugar-free hard candy around if you need something.

18. **If munching while you cook is a problem for you, try to prepare several meals at once to decrease the amount of time you will be vulnerable.**

19. **Keep healthy snacking alternatives available, such as sugar-free hard candies, sugar-free popsicles, or sugar-free flavored gelatin.**

20. **Always keep a bottle of water with you.** It will keep you feeling fuller between meals and is very healthy.

21. **Always have an escape route.** Do not put yourself in a situation where you feel unable to control your eating. If you find yourself overwhelmed at any time, have a plan for how you will allow yourself to leave.

22. **Monitor your progress.** Assess your body mass index (BMI) on a weekly or monthly basis. Weigh yourself weekly. Keep track of your workouts. Many people have difficulty when they stop monitoring themselves. We tend to feel more responsible for eating and exercise when we have to be held accountable.

23. **Be aware of visual cues for eating.** Let's say someone puts donuts on a desk nearby you at work or there is a community candy bowl you pass by several times a day. A little snack here and there may feel like nothing, but it all adds up. Break the connection between eating and the cue. Move the donuts to another part of the office. Get rid of the candy dish. If you find your cue is being with a particular friend, then attempt to alter the connection by going to a movie instead of dinner.

24. **When you have a craving, try waiting for 10 minutes before you eat anything.** When you do not immediately respond to cravings, they tend to decrease in intensity. If you do this over time, the craved food will lose its strength and power over you.

Case Study

Stuart always had a bowl of ice cream after dinner. His usual routine was to move to the living room, turn on the television, and at the first commercial go to the kitchen for ice cream. When he tried to stop having ice cream after dinner in the past, he would go to the living room, watch TV, and at the first commercial he would feel extreme anxiety and anger and usually have the ice cream anyway to rid himself of these feelings. He began to think the ice cream was in charge. In just about every other diet he tried over the years, it was always the ice cream that turned out to be the problem. First he would have just a few bites per evening, then a small bowl, eventually his usual serving, and that of course led to quitting the diet altogether.

Stuart came to my office for help. He wanted to change, but it was just too difficult. He desperately wanted it to work this time, so before the surgery he was determined to control the problem. The environmental triggers were just too overwhelming for him. We came up with a plan to solve this problem.

First, he would not sit down to watch television after eating and instead would take the dog for a stroll after dinner. Second, he would make sure ice cream was not available so he could not cheat in a moment of extreme anxiety. No ice cream was allowed in his house. Third, he would learn anxiety reduction techniques, such as deep breathing and motivating self-talk, to help get him through the tough transition. Fourth, he would keep sugar-free popsicles on hand as an acceptable substitution. Fifth, he had enjoyed making model airplanes in the past and would start again so his hands would be busy while watching television.

Stuart reported a month later that it was indeed difficult, but he had been able to make the transition. This was the change he was most worried about, and when he was able to finally make it, he began to tackle other problems with similar success.

Chapter 8

Weight Maintenance

OBJECTIVES

1. Compare weight maintenance and weight loss
2. List two main components to successful lifelong weight maintenance
3. Describe the importance of self-monitoring in weight maintenance

Weight loss attempts are complicated by many factors. The media entices us with mouth-watering commercials and ads depicting young, fit, happy people having fun and eating bacon double cheeseburgers. These images make us want to eat. Food is the main event in most social events ranging from baseball games, to weddings, to dating. Our environment makes it very difficult to maintain weight loss after we achieve our weight goal and begin to eat more again.

When we are not eating or thinking about eating, we are often dieting, reading about dieting, or planning our next one. The diet business is thriving. There are hundreds of diets available, and most will help you lose weight. Very few will help you understand the value of weight maintenance. We all seem very good at being on diets and just as good at being off diets, but not very good at maintenance.

People lose weight all the time, but usually gain it back as soon as they stop the diet. Adding an extra 20 pounds in the process is common. It is poor post-diet maintenance that causes people to gain the weight back. For those of you considering this surgery, maintenance has to be your ultimate goal. You will lose weight if you follow the diet after surgery, but maintenance is a lifelong challenge even for bariatric patients. Many people do gain some or all the weight back after surgery, so learning the proper steps in weight maintenance is very important.

PEOPLE LOSE WEIGHT ALL THE TIME but usually gain it back...Adding an extra 20 pounds in the process is common. It is poor post-diet maintenance that causes people to gain the weight back. For those of you considering this surgery, maintenance has to be your ultimate goal.

There is an incredibly strong pull to go back to our old eating habits. They are comfortable and familiar, and they just feel right. The habits are forged over many years. Think of your old eating habits as your default settings. You will want to revert to those default settings when under stress or when you reach your weight loss goal. Weight maintenance means resisting those urges to slip back into old eating patterns. It is an ongoing process that may be difficult in the beginning, but as you learn and practice these techniques, they will become second nature to you. Over many months and years, you can adjust your default settings. Just because you may have gained the weight back before does not mean that you will again.

PSYCHOLOGICAL BASICS OF WEIGHT MAINTENANCE IN THAT "IN-BETWEEN" STATE

So you've lost the weight. Congratulations! You have been through some very difficult situations and have been successful. Now your focus has to shift to weight maintenance.

We have been conditioned to be either "on" or "off" a diet. This is called "all-or-nothing thinking." This type of thinking usually leads to yo-yo dieting as we continually go on and off diets, losing, gaining, and then losing weight again and again. We are comfortable trying to diet, and comfortable not dieting, but somewhat uneasy in that in-between state of maintenance. It is called the "in-between" state because you may eat a bit more, but must not revert to old eating habits. Your challenge is to develop a whole new mindset. It will become your new default setting. With this mindset, you will always be on a diet to some extent because you will always be watching your food intake.

With maintenance, the diet is less strict. You have some leeway in what you eat and can eat a few more calories, but do not think of yourself as being "off" the diet.

Long-term maintenance involves the following two major components:

1. Watching your food intake
2. Lifelong continuation of your exercise program.

Your program's dietitian and surgeon will provide information on your maintenance diet food choices. Watch out for the tendency to overeat. This is a time when some people really let down their guard, so be careful. Our tendency is to reach the goal and then go "off" the diet. How you handle this time is critical for long-term success.

The point at which you are reaching your weight goal is a dangerous time. This is when it is natural to start to feel like "everyone else." You see everyone else can eat fast food and skip the exercise. You will appear like everyone else on the outside, but you are not. Don't ever lose sight of that fact, or you will be in danger of slipping back into your old habits.

You should be exercising at least three times per week. I recommend five times or more if possible. Once you reach your goal weight and maintenance begins, you may feel the urge to stop exercising. This will put you at risk to gain weight back. Exercise must continue indefinitely in order to keep the weight off. It is a very important component to weight maintenance. If you experience a drop in motivation to continue exercising, be sure to reread the motivational section of this book and talk to a friend. If all else fails, please make an appointment with a psychologist.

When you get to the weight maintenance stage, you must also continue to watch your food intake. This book does not go into detail on the science of weight maintenance, but rather discusses the psychological techniques to help keep you on track. Most bariatric surgery candidates have not had success at maintenance and have usually lost and gained weight many times. You may think the most difficult part of weight loss was the surgery, but weight maintenance has its own set of challenges.

YOU WILL APPEAR LIKE EVERYONE ELSE on the outside, but you are not. Don't ever lose sight of that fact, or you will be in danger of slipping back into your old habits.

Psychologically, you feel like you have completed your task. The weight is off, you are feeling better, looking better, and have a better mental outlook. Expect your self-talk to go something like this: "I can afford to take a couple of weeks off from exercising now, just a short vacation. I deserve it. I'll start again in 10 days." Beware. You have just taken the first step to a complete exercise meltdown. Chances are slim that you will soon start again. Do not fall into this trap. It is difficult to really motivate yourself to start an exercise program, so don't ever let it stop. If you experience a stressful period in your life, just cut back to two workouts per week. When the crisis passes, go back to your usual three to five times per week.

✓ TO DO

1. **Come to terms with the fact that if you want to keep the weight off, exercise must become a permanent part of your life.** Like brushing your teeth or taking a shower, it is essential activity that is here to stay.

2. **Do not believe the excuses and self-talk you tell yourself in order to avoid exercise.** Taking time off is a red flag. Your task is to motivate yourself. Remember how far you have come, and don't let anything stand in the way of your exercise.

3. **For some, it is easier to be "on" or "off" a diet than being on a maintenance diet because you have more choices.** Get yourself under control if you notice that you are cheating too much. Relocate your "middle ground."

4. **Realize you will never eat like others again.** You are different and have special needs and considerations. Make peace with this, and you will feel less anxiety over your differences. Try to look at your uniqueness as a positive. After all, look where it got you.

5. **Keep your eye on the scale.** Weigh yourself weekly. If you notice a few pounds of weight gain, it may just be the time of day or expected fluctuations in weight. If you notice a trend over a couple of weeks, take action. Sit down and plan your meals and exercise and get back on track. Getting back to basics is usually a good place to start. This means

checking your environment for trigger foods and keeping your exercise consistent. Begin using your food and exercise logbooks again.

6. **Positive self-talk will be important for the rest of your life.** Tell yourself you are worth the time and that you will not backslide.

7. **As always, if you are unable to gain control or motivate yourself, please call a psychologist for help.** After thousands of dollars in medical care, and countless days and hours working toward your goal, do not jeopardize what you have accomplished. Call for help if you need it. Often it is just a few weeks of assistance and you will be back on top.

Chapter 9

Relapse Prevention

OBJECTIVES

1. Define relapse prevention in weight loss
2. Describe healthy thoughts for use after a "slip"
3. List steps in bariatric psychology Emergency First Aid Kit

Relapse prevention is a term used by psychologists to describe a new perspective for a common reaction. Think of how many times you may have been watching your diet, had a bad day, ate something you regretted, and then said, "Well, I have blown it now. I might as well have some ice cream, too." Human beings have a tendency to try to be perfect, and if we aren't, then we just go back to our old habits. We call this "all-or-nothing thinking." It just means we either watch our diets perfectly, or we don't watch at all. An important key to long-term weight maintenance is learning relapse prevention techniques. These allow you to stay on your diet even though you may have eaten something you regret. They teach you to ignore "all-or-nothing" thinking.

✓ TO DO

1. **Realize no one is perfect.** You are not a robot. Do not expect to be 100-percent adherent with your bariatric diet.

2. **When you do "slip," you then have a choice.** You can either revert to the old eating patterns of the past, and eventually begin to gain weight, or learn from the "slip." Ask yourself some questions: Why did it happen? What can I learn from it so I will not make this mistake in the future?

3. **Stop the thoughts that say, "I already blew it. I'll start again Monday."** Replace that thinking with, "I only ate one piece of candy. It was 300 calories. I will not let this ruin all my progress. I am in charge." Use positive self-talk to your advantage. It is easier to stop yourself after one or two slips than after letting go for weeks or months.

4. **Recognize that there is no end to a lifestyle change. It will go on forever.**

5. **Focus on the big picture.** In any lifestyle change, there is a general trend toward success, but there are hundreds of daily and weekly ups and downs.

Do not focus on the tiny ups and downs, but rather the big picture.

Try a new mindset. Take your thinking from "If this doesn't work, I'll just go back to my old habits," to "No matter what happens I will get back on the horse. I will be successful, and not let small slips keep me from my goal of lifelong good health and excellent quality of life." Lifestyle changes never end.

EMERGENCY FIRST AID KIT

There will be times when you completely fall off the wagon. You slip into your old, comfortable eating pattern and stop exercising. Perhaps it will be a family crisis, relocation, or major change in your job. When this happens, it is time to go BACK TO BASICS.

Basics of Your Emergency First Aid Kit:

1. Scrutinize your environment for obstacles, and take all trigger foods out of the house.

2. Commit to monitoring yourself until you feel confident:
     a. Weigh yourself weekly.
     b. Start a new food log.
     c. Start a new exercise log.

3. Exercise immediately to reestablish the habit.

4. Set up rewards for exercise.

5. Shop for healthy foods and snacks.

6. Use positive self-talk. Remember where you started.

7. Look at your habits and obstacles to success. Rearrange and prioritize.

8. Contact a local bariatric program for support groups and attend several meetings.

Almost everyone will experience these episodes. Your choice is always to continue down that path or to use your Emergency First Aid Kit.

Chapter 10

Relationships and How They May Change After Surgery

OBJECTIVES

1. Explain why sabotage is common in relationships after bariatric surgery
2. Identify reasons why couples having surgery together have twice the stress
3. List healthy ways to deal with negative reactions from family members

Most bariatric patients never consider the psychological effects of extreme weight loss on themselves and those around them. It is not uncommon for couples to divorce or break up after this surgery. This chapter will help you understand what kind of emotions and roadblocks you may face in your relationships. Spouses or significant others often have similar reactions after bariatric surgery. What is described here is normal human behavior and is no reflection on the quality of your relationship or the character of your partner.

Before surgery, you have equilibrium in your relationship and in your home environment. After surgery, these things will change drastically. If you change, your partner has to change in some ways as well. People do not really enjoy change, especially when it is not their decision or their surgery. When this happens, the partner may attempt to change the relationship back to the way it was when it was familiar, comfortable, and he or she knew what to expect.

SABOTAGE

The actions taken by a partner to restore familiar equilibrium often take the form of sabotage to the diet/exercise program. Your partner may give a subtle sigh when you go to exercise or complain about not going to a restaurant or even bring you your favorite food "because I knew you'd love it." I have heard stories of wives that suddenly begin baking or cooking mouth-watering meals that their husbands cannot eat. Most do not even realize that they are doing it and are embarrassed when it is brought to their attention. If you notice this kind of behavior, talk to your partner. He or she is probably dealing with many feelings he or she does not feel comfortable expressing. A good conversation about how weight loss is affecting your family members usually helps.

COUPLES HAVING BARIATRIC SURGERY TOGETHER

It happens more and more often: Two people will have bariatric surgery together. It is difficult being the patient. It can also be trying for the significant other. When couples have the surgery together, it can be twice as hard. Each person has the problems of both the

THE ACTIONS TAKEN BY A PARTNER to restore familiar equilibrium often take the form of sabotage to the diet/exercise program.

patient and the significant other. I have found that people in healthy relationships do well together, but those having problems often see increased relationship difficulties after surgery. If you plan to have the surgery with a partner, try to remain independent as far as exercise and food choices. Working out together is a bonus, but do not get into the habit of skipping workouts because your partner cannot participate. Do not let your partner be in charge of your habits.

Good communication is the key to couples' success. Before the surgery, discuss the logistics of the changes you must make. After the surgery, talk to each other weekly about your feelings regarding the surgery and the changes you are both experiencing. It is possible to grow much closer as a couple as a result of this experience.

There will be a tendency to talk each other into tiny cheats. Typically, this is how it works: "C'mon, let's just have a little bit. We deserve it." Having the surgery together represents some increased challenges, but has the potential for increased excitement and support. Keep communication flowing and problems will be minimized.

✓ TO DO

There is a natural human tendency to want to try to put things back the way they were. This includes spouses and significant others. We are comfortable in our old habits. Often family members do not realize they have subconscious motives for bringing "cheat" foods into the house. Underneath the surface, they crave the old, comfortable habits of the past. If this occurs in your home, try having everyone talk about how they are doing with all the changes. Keeping the lines of communication open is the key. I recommend that my patients ask their significant others how they are doing every few weeks.

Often there is a common fear underlying the sabotage. The spouse or partner feels that the patient is going to lose weight and leave him or her for someone else. This thinking may seem ridiculous, but chances are pretty good that your partner may have already joked about it. You may even joke that you will do it. The problem is that he or she is not really joking. It is a fear that drives people to sabotage their partner's efforts. If the lines of communication are closed, relationships are at a real risk of failing.

As you lose weight quickly after the surgery, it can be difficult to get used to your new body. It can be just as difficult for those around you. They may be very proud and happy for you, but they may also have a hard time adjusting to the changes. Bariatric surgery is almost as difficult for the family as it is for the patient.

OTHER REACTIONS FROM FAMILY MEMBERS..."LET ME JUST POINT OUT..."

Another common emotion felt by family members is fear that the patient will somehow hurt him- or herself. I hear, "She's not eating enough protein," and "He's not exercising," and "He's not chewing enough" often from family members. The family member is usually very worried about the wellbeing of the patient. He or she shows concern by constantly reminding the patient of what he or she should be doing. This constant friction can affect the relationship. I advise family members to make a serious effort not to do this. The patient has been through psychological assessment and is able to understand the requirements of diet and exercise. It will ultimately be up to him or her to take responsibility for his or her own behavior. Constant "reminding" only serves to alienate the patient and cause stress in the

AS YOU LOSE WEIGHT QUICKLY after the surgery, it can be difficult to get used to your new body. It can be just as difficult for those around you. They may be very proud and happy for you, but they may also have a hard time adjusting to the changes.

relationship. The relationship will improve if each person understands what the other is feeling and makes an effort to stop the behavior that aggravates the relationship.

"YOU'RE TAKING THE EASY WAY OUT"

It is a natural tendency for people to attribute their own successes to intelligence, character, or hard work, and the successes of others to luck. So it is not uncommon to hear statements like, "He's taking the easy way out. He had bariatric surgery." This is, for the most part, a misguided attitude. People think it's easy because they are seduced by the drastic before and after pictures they see in the media. The truth is that almost everyone having bariatric surgery will lose weight, and lose it much more quickly than on any diet. This is the primary reason why so many think of it as the latest "I gotta try it" diet. I have met people who were only 65 pounds overweight, with no serious health problems, who actually tried to gain more weight so they would be eligible for the surgery. The surgery is often mistakenly viewed as the latest diet craze, or an easy, foolproof way to lose weight.

It is the fastest way to lose weight, but it is anything but easy. Living with the aftermath of surgery may include sickness and unpleasant-looking physical changes. Your world as you know it will change, and you will be faced with having to exercise for the rest of your life. It is rare, but some people die from bariatric surgery, and others may end up with complications that land them back in the hospital again and again. The important thing to know is the psychology behind those who may try to talk you down. They may have struggled with their own weight and are looking to strike out at someone who has had tremendous success. Understand why they do it, and do not let it affect your success.

ANGER

Anger and resentment on the part of the family is a common occurrence at some point after surgery. The family is asked to make changes at home, worry about the life and health of the patient, and put up with some intense mood swings. As one of my patients explained, "It was my choice to have this surgery, but my family was drafted." The family may resent having to deal with the obesity issue in the first place. Even if they are supportive and loving, they may perceive that your

Case Study

Theresa's family was very supportive of her weight loss. She had been over 400 pounds, and the rest of her family had body weights in the normal range. As she began to lose weight, she received much reinforcement from family members. After several months, her mother jokingly asked her to stop losing weight "before you get smaller than I am." This request was upsetting to her, and she brought it up in group therapy. The group members advised her to talk to her mother about it. She was afraid of alienating her mother with continued weight loss.

obesity is due to a lack of prior action. I have heard patients' family members say, "This is unfair. I have been exercising all my life, but now I have to deal with this because he refused to exercise for 25 years. It is not right." This is a normal reaction, and should pass with time. Encourage your family to tell you how they feel. If it does not improve, the problem runs deeper, and you should consider family counseling.

ABUSE

Some spouses will use weight as an excuse to abuse. They may make negative remarks, threaten to leave the relationship, withhold affection, and blame it all on the weight. This is considered emotional abuse. For some, it may even escalate to physical abuse. A person on the receiving end in this situation is likely to feel powerless, have low self esteem, and after weight loss, may decide to leave the relationship. If this describes you, leaving may be your best option. No one should endure physical or emotional abuse. At the very least, couples therapy should be undertaken.

OTHERS CONCERNED WITH YOUR WEIGHT

There are those mothers, fathers, or friends that have spent years telling you to lose weight. These are the ones that say, "Do you really think you should eat that extra helping?" They make comments about other people's weight around you and seem to have made it a hobby to point out your weight.

It is a strange phenomenon that when you do lose weight, often this same person starts to discuss how thin you are becoming or how you should "fatten up a little bit." For these people, it is difficult to stop talking about your weight because it has become a habit.

Well-meaning family members may also say things like, "You were so fat, you were gigantic. We all talked about it and didn't know what to do." They may unwittingly say things that hurt your feelings. Discuss their comments with them. They may not realize what they are saying or how it may make you feel.

Your weight loss may change others' perceptions of themselves. For example, if you are 5'6" and walk into a room full of professional basketball players, you will perceive yourself as being short. If you walk into a kindergarten classroom, you will feel tall. Your weight loss will have psychological effects on those around you as well as yourself.

Common Reactions to Weight Loss

There are many kinds of changes that can occur when one begins to lose weight after bariatric surgery. No one person experiences all of these changes, but most will encounter several of them.

"WHEN I LOOK IN A MIRROR I AM SHOCKED"

Almost everyone has this reaction to rapid weight loss. It takes time, and perhaps years, for your mental representation of yourself to match your new body dimensions. It is not uncommon to catch a glimpse of your reflection in a window or mirror and be shocked at what you see. When you are going about your daily business, your mind forgets what you have accomplished.

THE BODY CHANGES RAPIDLY, but the emotions change much more slowly.

With time you will come to terms with it. Some people adjust quickly, and others take years. Some may never have a realistic mental picture of themselves, especially if they spent most of their life being overweight. Even overweight, people often do not have an accurate body image. Most recall shock at seeing photos of themselves and saying, "I didn't realize I had gained that much weight." Body image disparity is very common, especially in females.

There is both a physical and an emotional component to body image. The body changes rapidly, but the emotions change much more slowly. Expect it to take some time, even years. I advise my patients to think of it as a novelty. Your mental interpretation of the experience will play a part in determining if it is a minor annoyance or a major problem. If you interpret it as a minor annoyance, it will have less of an impact on you. Patience is the cure, and eventually your mental self will more closely coincide with your physical self.

One technique for learning to appreciate your true size/body image is to look at yourself in the mirror and find at least five things you like about your body. It could be your wrists, your calves, your neck, or even your fingers. Another technique is to look at photos of yourself at various stages of weight loss. Do not avoid the camera during this transition. It will help you stay in touch with your actual size.

If for some reason your body image disparity does not resolve on its own, it may be necessary to attend some groups, talk to other patients, or talk to a psychologist about the problem. The negative messages some people receive throughout their lives do not magically dissipate after weight loss and can interfere with having a more accurate body image.

FEELING CONFIDENT

With confidence, you can walk into a room without feeling as though people think you are fat. You will feel free to be yourself without worrying about how you look. This newfound feeling may translate into taking more chances with your life. Perhaps you will find new relationships, a new career, a new sport, or other new challenges. Your confidence will increase with each success as you learn to take control. You begin to replace "I can't" with "I can." Confidence is a wonderful feeling, and your assignment is to enjoy it. Use it to achieve your goals, whatever they may be.

FEELINGS OF ACCOMPLISHMENT

You did it! You have been through so much and you are winning! Other problems may appear smaller by comparison. This feeling helps keep you motivated to continue with your diet and exercise program. Perhaps you have been setting goals and achieving rewards. This serves to increase your feeling of accomplishment.

There are no expected ways to behave or change after bariatric surgery. Do not feel pressured to make sweeping changes in your life to live up to other people's expectations. Be kind to yourself, and move at your own pace. But do not be surprised if after your recent success, you choose to tackle other issues in your life.

FEELING NORMAL

For the first time in ages, your weight is in the normal range and you feel less self-conscious. You feel like you fit in. You can shop in regular stores in the mall, and others can buy clothes for you. You can fit into rides at theme parks and in airplane seats. Your weight no longer sets you apart, and this feeling can be comforting and exhilarating. Congratulations!

FEELING LESS HELPLESS

After trying one diet after another, many people begin to feel helpless over their weight. Over time, that feeling of helplessness can expand to other areas of your life, such as career, relationships, health, or even your future. Another effect of weight loss is feeling an increased sense of control and a decreased sense of helplessness. This is an empowering feeling as you realize your future is in your own hands. Again, enjoy the feeling. Feeling in control is a powerful emotion that can open up a world of opportunities for you.

FOCUSING ON OTHER PEOPLE'S WEIGHT

You've seen it many times. The ex-smoker who can't stop talking about smoking or pointing out other people's smoking. They may dramatically gag and cough at the sight of a smoker. A similar fixation can also occur in people who lose a large amount of weight. The formerly overweight person becomes obsessed with other people's weight and urges others to do what they did. They may even comment on overweight people they see or offer "well-meaning" advice just as others did to them. This person is excited about all the changes he or she has made, and it seems that all they can talk about is weight loss. On the other hand, this behavior can be distasteful and disturbing to others around them and can even serve to alienate old friends.

> **FEELING IN CONTROL** is a powerful emotion that can open up a world of opportunities for you.

Excitement about your success is a good thing, but monitor yourself and be aware of the reactions of others. If you have a tendency to be this way, be aware that many an old friendship have disintegrated due to this kind of obsession.

"MY FRIENDS ARE JEALOUS OF MY WEIGHT LOSS"

The possibility exists that some people will be jealous of your weight loss, especially if you previously enjoyed eating out together or dining at each other's homes. You may all have enjoyed food without having thought about its connection to weight. Perhaps the subject of weight was ignored because you were all in the same boat. But now you have not only changed the dynamic of the group, you have shined a light on the subject of weight. These friends may now feel uncomfortable around you because you have succeeded, especially if they have attempted weight loss themselves. Talk to them about how you feel, and listen openly to their feelings. Voicing your concerns can begin to alleviate them, or in some situations, it just takes time for them to get used to the changes. It is your right to discuss anything you like, but try to keep the conversation on subjects you enjoyed prior to weight loss. There will be fewer problems if everyone involved feel as though nothing has really changed.

Case Study

Stephanie did very well after bariatric surgery. One year after the surgery, she had lost over 150 pounds. She went to the gym almost every day. She was truly a success story. One day I received a frantic phone call. She was angry and said, "All of my friends are jealous of my weight loss." She complained that she was not being invited to activities because of this jealousy. We talked for a while, and it became apparent that she was engaging in certain behaviors that were driving her friends away. She was urging them all to lose weight, and they felt uncomfortable being around their friend because of her inability to discuss subjects other than food or weight. Going out to dinner as they had in the past had become a trying experience for everyone. We came up with a plan. She understood that it was her enthusiasm that was exciting and motivating her to talk about weight and weight loss, but that perhaps it was uncomfortable for those around her to hear. She decided to try to change her interactions with her friends to include subjects other than food and weight loss, and she called several weeks later to say that her relationships with her friends had indeed improved, and they had not been jealous, just bored and uncomfortable.

Now and then Stephanie comes to a support group. She says her relationships are doing well, and she often counsels others in the group to watch their conversations with friends.

CHANGING YOUR LIFE

Rapid weight loss can be exciting. The first year or so after the surgery can be life-changing. Not only are you changing physically, but you are changing emotionally as well. Emotions tend to be very strong that first year, and people sometimes get caught up in the excitement. I recommend not making any major life changes during this first year. Give your emotions time to reach an equilibrium. Try to focus on your health and habits for the first year, and save the big decisions, such as marriage, divorce, or having children, for several months down the road.

CHANGING YOUR STYLE OF DRESS

Admit it. You have dreamed about it, fantasized about it, and you are ready to wear what you want and have fun with your clothes. You may find your style of dress has completely changed, often becoming a bit more trendy or more provocative. The thought of

Case Study

Lina had been overweight all her life. Before surgery she said, "I can't imagine what it will be like when I actually have a normal weight." After surgery, she lost over 120 pounds in about six months. She was excited, people were relating to her in a completely different way, and she lost perspective. Although she had been married for over 20 years, she met a man on the Internet, and sight unseen, moved to Italy to live with him. She would not be talked out of it or convinced to wait. About five months later she returned, and wanted her old life back again now that she had a more realistic perspective. She was luckily able to reestablish the relationship with her husband, but not all spouses are that understanding. It is always a good idea to give drastic changes some time.

being able to wear what we want often helps to keep us on our diet and exercise program. However, some people take it to the extreme. I sometimes get calls from family members who complain, "She's gone off the deep end and wears tube tops and mini skirts." Whatever your clothing choice, be aware that others are watching you and may be concerned with the changes. Consider talking about it with those who have difficulty with the "new you." Your clothing choice is yours alone to make, and you deserve to enjoy yourself after all your hard work.

At the other end of the spectrum, some feel there must be something wrong with them because they do not want to wear tight-fitting clothes. They feel more comfortable in loose fitting clothes. This too is normal. Try not to let others' expectations influence your choices. There is no right or wrong way to dress. What is right for you is right.

"I'M THIN, BUT I STILL FEEL DIFFERENT THAN OTHER PEOPLE"

You may feel "different" for some time. After all, you are different. You have a tiny stomach and do not have the same food choices you had in the past. You have gone through drastic lifestyle, physical, and psychological changes. Yes, you are different, but that will be a positive or negative depending on your perspective.

✓ TO DO

1. Tell yourself it is O.K. to feel like you are different.
2. Concentrate on the positives and everything you have gained.

3. Ask yourself, "Am I better off now than I was before?"

FEAR OF WEIGHT GAIN

A large percentage of patients experience an intense fear of regaining their weight. For many, they have experienced what they consider to be a miracle. Often after a lifelong battle with weight, they have won, but the nagging question is "How long will I be able to keep it off?" This feeling is normal when you think about the yo-yo dieting that most patients have gone through. History tells us that excitement over weight loss is almost always replaced by sadness and disgust over weight gain. It is no wonder we fear the return of weight, even after bariatric surgery.

If you follow the diet and continue to exercise for life, you will most likely not gain the weight back. You should expect to gain a little back eventually. This is considered normal. But if you follow the diet and continue to exercise for life, you should feel confident that you can keep it off. Let the knowledge that you and only you have the power to keep it off and be a motivator to stick with it. Even with this knowledge, some people will react in an unhealthy way. Here are a few examples:

A. Hypervigilance. This reaction is one of precision. If a person is supposed to eat two ounces of chicken, then they make absolutely sure they are not eating 2.1 ounces. A patient of mine would focus on eating the exact amount of food she was allotted, and not one bit more. Going over the allotted amount would cause a very negative effect. She would become sad, withdrawn, guilty, and anxious. She would follow this with an extra 45-minute workout to "compensate" for the lapse.

Over time, this reaction tends to become more extreme. Not only is it difficult to be so precise, but it can drive others crazy. Also, it makes very little difference in overall weight loss and weight maintenance. As with other psychological reactions, the first step is becoming aware of the behavior. The next step is to attempt to change it. If you are unable to change the behavior on your own, seek help from a psychologist for a few weeks to overcome the reaction. A trained professional can usually help you to get the behavior under control fairly quickly.

B. Purging. Purging is self-induced vomiting. There are people with no history of purging who suddenly start after surgery. The root of this problem is fear of weight gain, coupled with an inability to control emotional eating patterns.

Purging is a full-fledged eating disorder. If you have never purged, do not try it. If you are now purging, you are putting your health in serious jeopardy and must stop immediately. Ask for professional help if you are unable to stop on your own.

Take note of these warning signs. If you are in the habit of taking a bite, chewing it up, then spitting it out, you could be taking the first steps toward a dangerous eating disorder. It may eventually progress to swallowing and purging. An eating disorder is just as devastating to your health and wellbeing as obesity, so don't fool yourself.

C. Eating too few calories for good health. This reaction is one of "if a little is good, then even less will be better." You will already be highly restricted in the amount of calories per day you are able to consume. A person with this reaction will start to eat even less. It is not a hard habit to get into since you already will not be very hungry. Less is not more in the case of bariatric

Case Study

Charlotte had unrealistic hopes for the surgery. She thought she would not be tempted to eat her favorite foods or if she did that she would be satisfied with a bite or two. Unfortunately, she soon found she battled the same urges to eat she had always experienced in the past. She was unable to stop herself from eating the foods she has always loved, and discovered that she could "undo the damage" by purging. Charlotte had never used purging as a means to control weight prior to surgery. She admitted this in a monthly support group for bariatric patients.

She told me it started because she felt she had too much to lose if she ate what she liked, so she purged. She said, "I never lost this much weight before, and I'm so scared of going backward again." This behavior is very difficult to stop, and the health ramifications can be catastrophic. It took months of very hard work in therapy to solve the problem.

patients. It is difficult to get enough nutrition after surgery, but restricting it even further can have very negative effects on your health.

If you find yourself in this category, know that the longer you continue the behavior, the more difficult it will be to stop. Know also that weight loss after surgery is rapid even with the recommended diet. If you are unable to stop on your own, seek the help of a professional as soon as possible. This is the equivalent of an eating disorder and can be dangerous to your health.

Often it is the family that brings this problem to the attention of the patient. They worry about the amount of food intake and possibly the unhealthy physical appearance of the patient and decide confrontation is the answer. You may not even realize there is a problem until confronted. If this happens, please listen to their concerns, and realize your perspective on food might not be realistic.

This surgery requires a change in perspective about dieting. On regular diets, the thinking is the less you eat, the more you lose. After bariatric surgery, the thinking must change to "I'll lose quickly and remain healthy by filling my pouch with high quality proteins." Rapid weight loss without following your prescribed diet is not healthy, and it is possible to end up back in the hospital with complications. You now require the high octane food your body craves. Nourish it well. Follow the program guidelines and you will lose the weight.

WHY DO I FEEL ANGER?

Patients do not usually expect to feel angry a couple of months after surgery, but it is more common than most people think. Let's face it— overweight people often are treated badly in our society. They are called names, pointed at, laughed at, discriminated against, and, as a result, usually have low self esteem because of this. There seems to be a perception in the general population that weight loss surgery is an "easy out," and prejudice against overweight people in our society is still accepted. Unfortunately, if you hear that obese people are lazy, unmotivated, and have no willpower, over time you are likely to start believing these labels yourself.

When someone is disrespectful to you as an obese person, you may be angry and may even come to expect it. When you lose weight, people may begin to treat you differently. You may be treated with more respect. This may unexpectedly bring out feelings of anger in some

Case Study

Stephanie lost over 100 pounds with the surgery, and ended up being a size 10. As a business executive, she said she had always been considered "competent and intelligent," but after her weight loss she was considered "a piece of meat" by the men in the company. She was highly disturbed by this change in reaction of men, and looked for reasons to avoid interactions with men outside of work. Weight can allow a person to be sexually invisible for the most part. Weight loss may take away the sexual barrier and may be uncomfortable to some patients.

patients because you are still the same person you always were. The only thing that has changed is the outside. Patients tell me, "I should be happy someone whistled at me today, but instead I just feel sad and angry."

This is only a stage in your weight loss journey, and you will pass through it. Be patient with yourself and patient with people in general. Again, it is human nature to judge a book by its cover to some extent. You are just sporting a new cover. My patients tell me it is a phase, and eventually you will become more accepting of the reactions of others. The challenge is not to isolate yourself or withdraw from others because of this feeling.

The bottom line is that others' perceptions of us have an effect on how we see ourselves. Just as the label of "lazy" has an effect when one is obese, the label of "piece of meat" can have an effect as well. Never forget that your personality, your qualities, and your value as a human being remain no matter what size you are.

RETURN TO OLD HABITS TO PLEASE OTHERS

Many patients have sad stories from their past. Maybe they include a dominating family member who rejects them after weight loss. There may be a subconscious urge to regain weight in order to regain acceptance with this person. This is a dangerous situation and should be handled in individual therapy. Often the patient does not know why he or she is regaining the weight. It is not a problem with your weight that alienates you from the person, but a problem within that person. Thankfully this is not a very common occurrence, but it is serious and requires professional help.

"I CAN'T BE FINISHED LOSING ALL THE WEIGHT"

It is not uncommon to hear a patient say, "The doctor told me I am at goal weight, but I think he's wrong." There is so much positive reinforcement from weight loss that it is often difficult to admit you have achieved the goal after years of trying. The reluctance or inability to accept that the maintenance stage has been reached is extremely difficult for some patients. A person may spend years trying to lose weight and then more time getting the surgery and going through everything involved. When your goal weight is finally achieved, it can be difficult after that tremendous effort to shift your focus to something else. Weight loss can become like a drug, and the reactions of others can become addicting.

✓ TO DO

Come to terms with the fact that thinking about weight loss has been an all-consuming passion, but that now it is time to look beyond the weight. It is OK to add some foods back into your diet. You did it! It is time to enjoy all those things you had in mind when you went for the surgery. Your job will never be completely finished though, because you must still concentrate on the maintenance of lifelong exercise and a healthy diet. This is a time to test different foods and explore your new mobility and outlook. You have earned the right to enjoy yourself.

> **COME TO TERMS** with the fact that thinking about weight loss has been an all-consuming passion, but that now it is time to look beyond the weight.

The most important thing to remember about all of these possible emotional changes is to keep the lines of communication open with your friends, family, and coworkers. Do not be afraid to enlist the help of a professional when necessary. Welcome and encourage feedback about the new you. You can learn from each other if you keep an open mind.

"I THOUGHT ALL MY PROBLEMS WOULD GO AWAY AFTER I LOST WEIGHT"

It is easy to look at before and after photos and think, "She sure seems happy. No problems can be big problems when you look like that." Realistically, people have problems no matter what they weigh. Whether it be relationship conflicts, bills, health issues, anxiety, or anything else, weight loss is not the answer. People who magically expect happiness with weight loss are often shocked and disappointed that many of their problems still exist.

This can be a difficult time for some patients. It is easy to attribute almost all of our problems to weight before surgery, but to what do we attribute them after weight loss? Losing weight can provide many incredible benefits, but guaranteed happiness is not one of them. If you are in this category, it would be very helpful to go to therapy for a few months. With the help of a psychologist and/or some support groups, you can work toward sorting out your problems and hopefully finding some of that elusive happiness.

Chapter 12

Depression After Surgery

OBJECTIVES
1. List symptoms of depression
2. Identify actions to take if feeling depressed
3. List possible reasons for depression after bariatric surgery

L ife after bariatric surgery will be different. How it differs will vary from person to person. Some patients will become depressed after surgery. This section will help you learn to identify symptoms of depression and how to help yourself.

You might say, "I can't imagine being depressed when losing weight." Believe it or not, this happens frequently. When people go through surgery and/or drastic lifestyle changes, depression can be a side effect. I have seen patients who previously had a tendency to become depressed react to the stress of surgery by falling into a depressive episode.

HOW DO I KNOW IF I'M DEPRESSED?

The majority of bariatric patients will not become depressed following surgery. Some will become mildly depressed and some severely depressed. It is important to be able to recognize the symptoms of depression, so you may ask for help if indicated.

Symptoms of depression:

1. **Sadness.** A depressed person does not have to be sad all the time. Feeling sad most of the time or most of the days per week is enough.

2. **Loss of interest.** A depressed person does not look forward to events or activities anymore. This person may have liked going to the theater for example, but now it sounds like more trouble than it is worth.

3. **Changes in sleep habits.** A depressed person may feel very tired and sleep more hours than usual, or may find themselves sleeping less than usual. For example, this person may find it difficult to get to sleep, and then wake up very early in the morning without being able to go back to sleep. Sleep apnea can influence your answer to this question.

4. **Changes in appetite.** For some, food may not look appetizing and food intake will decrease. For

others, hunger is a constant and they will be more focused on food. It is not uncommon for a person to gain weight from an increased appetite due to depression and then blame the depression on the weight gain. For these people, treatment usually results in weight loss. Bariatric surgery may influence this symptom because you may not feel hungry.

5. **Social isolation.** You may look for reasons to stay home and not see your friends. You may cancel activities with others because of a headache or tell them you have to do a chore. When a person is depressed, her world will shrink. She often sees fewer people, engages in fewer activities, and spends more time alone at home. This just serves to increase the depression.

6. **Helplessness.** A depressed person will begin to feel that he has no control over the events in his life. He often feel like a victim, and that there is no action he can take that will alleviate the pain and suffering or fix the problem.

7. **Hopelessness.** Often a depressed person will feel as though there is no hope for the future, or she can't see herself ever feeling better. To her, it seems like sadness will follow her forever.

8. **Worthlessness.** Some people talk about the overwhelming feeling of worthlessness that sometimes accompanies depression. It is common for this person to isolate further, and ignore offers from others for help. He is, after all, "not worth the trouble."

9. **Irritability.** Usually a depressed person will feel more irritable and easily angered. She may be quick to jump to negative conclusions about others. A family member may be the first to bring it to her attention, but an irritable person may not be ready to hear this news.

10. **Low motivation.** You may find it difficult to get through your "to do" list for the day. You may have to force yourself to take care of your usual chores, routines, self-care, and activities.

11. **Suicidal ideation.** This is the most dangerous symptom of all. If you are contemplating suicide or have said to yourself, "Things would be better if I wasn't around," then your situation is extreme. It is imperative that you get help immediately.

If you have several of the symptoms listed above, it is important to get help, especially if it is affecting your work or relationships. Depression can be alleviated. Without treatment, most depression will usually decrease on its own in about six months, but do not wait. Untreated depression makes it difficult to stick to lifestyle changes and may lead to problems with weight loss or maintenance. Get the professional help you need as soon as you realize you have a problem.

With the assistance of professionals, depression can be decreased or even alleviated in weeks or a short period of time. State-of-the-art treatment for depression involves both antidepressants and talk therapy. Research continues to show that these two treatments together are the best and fastest way to decrease depressive symptoms. The most important advice is to see someone if you feel depressed. There is help.

For a prescription for an antidepressant, you may seek the expertise of a psychiatrist. The psychiatrist will prescribe the antidepressant that is most useful

> **WITHOUT TREATMENT,** most depression will usually decrease on its own in about six months, but do not wait. Untreated depression makes it difficult to stick to lifestyle changes and may lead to problems with weight loss or maintenance.

for people with symptoms similar to yours. Most psychiatrists do not do talk therapy. Some people prefer to use their PCP (primary care physician) to prescribe an antidepressant, but some PCPs are reluctant to do this. Whichever route you choose, understand that antidepressants take from 3 to 6 weeks to work, and there will be side effects. Discuss the specifics with the doctor that prescribes for you.

For talk therapy, you should seek the expertise of a psychologist, social worker, or mental health counselor. You should likely do what is called cognitive/behavioral therapy. This treatment works with your thought patterns and behaviors to alleviate depression and has been shown in research to work well.

If you are thinking about suicide, this is very serious. When one is depressed, suicide can seem like a solution, but it is the depression itself that causes this skewed thinking. I have worked with many patients that became suicidal, but months later when the depression was alleviated, they said, "Thank goodness I didn't do it. It seemed like a way out at the time." If this describes you, you must call for help immediately. Talk to a family member, call a professional, or call 911 if it is an emergency. You do not have to feel depressed. There is help.

WHEN ONE IS DEPRESSED, suicide may seem like a solution, but it is the depression itself that causes this skewed thinking.

Depression can come from many different sources. Some of these sources are the following:

1. **Mourning the loss of food.** Food has always been there as a way to help you cope with emotions. After bariatric surgery, you may feel like you are on the outside looking in, especially when socializing or in restaurants. This mourning period is normal and will usually subside with time.

2. **Depression can come from the reactions you receive from family, coworkers, spouses, and even strangers.** The reactions of others

may be positive or negative, but the change itself may lead to depression as you begin to alter your self-image.

3. **Those that have a history of depression may become depressed due to the stress of life after surgery.**

4. **Those that had unrealistic expectations that weight loss would make them happy are at risk for depression.**

5. **It is common for people focused on weight to base their mood on the number on the scale.** If the number on the scale is up, mood becomes depressed. If the number on the scale goes down, mood becomes happy. Do not fall into that trap. Weight will normally fluctuate depending on many physical factors throughout the day, week, or month. Do not let your mood be dictated by a number on the scale. I recommend choosing a range based on your goal and normal fluctuations. For example, if your weight goal is 150, choose a realistic weight range of 150 to 160. Weigh yourself weekly. As long as your weight stays within this range, you are OK. If it exceeds this range, you need to make some changes. Refer to the Emergency First Aid section in this book, if necessary.

Chapter 13

Is It True That Some People Do Not Lose Very Much Weight After Surgery?

OBJECTIVES

1. List categories of patients that have difficulty sustaining weight loss after surgery
2. Describe action to take if not losing weight as expected

There are several categories of patients who may experience some psychological problems related to food after surgery. Listed in the upcoming pages are some of the problems that have been reported. If any of these apply to you, you should make an appointment as soon as possible with a psychologist by calling the 800 number on the back of your insurance card or consulting with your bariatric program's psychologist. Most of these

problems can be helped if professionals are
consulted early.

THE UNCONTROLLED EMOTIONAL EATER

This person has not addressed the reasons why he
eats and consumes food "automatically" out of habit or
when bored, stressed, or sad. The first six months
after surgery, a person may lose weight even while
eating in this way, but eventually the weight loss will
stop and he or she will begin to gain it back. If he or
she is in a bariatric support group, he or she will
realize others are losing weight and he or she is not
losing as much. Everyone I speak to before the surgery
is convinced they will be able to handle the drastic
change in a lifelong pattern of eating behavior, but
unfortunately this is not always the case. If you see
yourself in this scenario, please contact a psychologist.
In sessions, you will examine thoughts and triggers
that are associated with this emotional eating, and you
will learn many techniques to put you back in control.

THE VICTIM OF ABUSE

Too many people in our society are sexually,
physically, and/or emotionally abused as children. A
traumatic past can have an effect on a person's life for
many years, even if he or she is unaware of the impact.
For a small percentage of victims, weight serves the
unconscious purpose of protection. It is usually a
feeling as opposed to an articulated thought, but it can
affect a patient's ability to lose weight after surgery.
These victims may subconsciously use weight to feel
tougher, to make themselves unattractive, or to keep
people at a physical or emotional distance. It is not
unusual for a victim of abuse to experience a drastic
slowdown in weight loss several months after surgery.

They report experiencing feelings of vulnerability, anxiety, or feeling unsafe. The usual psychological reaction is to eat a little bit too much, so weight loss stops, and the uncomfortable feelings cease. This is understandable behavior under the circumstances. It is extremely uncomfortable and frightening for someone to lose that safety cocoon.

If you have an abuse history, it does not mean you will experience this. It is not a universal reaction to abuse, and there are multiple reasons why a person has a weight problem. But if you notice you have a couple of months with no significant weight loss, this may be
a reason.

These feelings can be controlled, but therapy is required. In therapy, you can learn to deal with the anxiety caused by the weight loss. Within several weeks, most people are feeling stronger, in control, and are then able to continue with the program.

THE BINGE EATER

Binge eating can be understood as eating more food than most people would eat in a certain amount of time or in a certain situation. The most important aspect to binge eating is the feeling of being out of control. Binge eaters do not necessarily make themselves vomit after eating. There is usually a feeling of shame, guilt, or disgust after binging.

Binge eating is considered a risky behavior. If you binge before surgery, you will likely experience an urge to binge after surgery. Stress, difficult relationships, life changes, and even dieting can lead to an increase in episodes. After surgery, it is difficult to eat large quantities, so some people become frequent snackers or "grazers."

Case Study

Joshua had a problem with binge eating. At the age of 28, he had been binging for five years. When his weight reached 300 pounds, he decided to have bariatric surgery. At his pre-surgery psychological appointment, he did not disclose that he was binging, and his surgery was scheduled. Two years later after reaching 175 pounds, he began to regain weight. When his weight reached 240 pounds, he came to my office for help.

It took almost six months of weekly therapy and hard work for Joshua to gain control over his eating. He said he was embarrassed by the binging, did most of his eating in secret, and did not want to tell anyone before the surgery. He was certain that the surgery would "cure" him of the problem. He said, "I thought because I would be losing weight I would be motivated to stop, but it didn't work."

Joshua checks in every now and then. He told me binging is still an issue, but he wins most of the time. He has been able to lose 200 pounds and keep it off for a year.

Binging is considered an eating disorder. Binging/grazing has been associated with weight regain after surgery, so it is important to learn to control this behavior. An eating disorder specialist can help you. Choose a psychologist familiar with eating disorders. You may also be directed to a psychiatrist for an evaluation for an antidepressant.

Binge eating is treatable and controllable with help. Start with a group and/or individual therapy. Only you know if you feel out of control with your eating, so if necessary, please ask for assistance.

THE UNREALISTIC PATIENT

Some people come into bariatric surgery with the expectation that it will magically force them to rigidly follow a diet. If they have been unable to follow a diet in the past, they may also have difficulty after surgery. These people may decide that it does not matter if they follow the diet because they have the same impulses to cheat that they have always had. At some point they regret having the surgery and may

Case Study

Alberto had his jaw wired shut 20 years ago. He lost to his goal weight, but as soon as the wires were removed he went right back to his old eating habits and regained all the weight. Ten years ago, he had a bariatric procedure. Again, he lost the weight, but regained it all within two years. Alberto was always looking for something external (surgery, wires) to stop him from eating. He came to me wanting another bariatric surgery. From his history, it was clear he would need help in order to be successful with keeping the weight off. Alberto came to therapy for three months, during which time he focused on all the thoughts, behaviors, and excuses he had used most of his life. With practice, and by learning to control anxiety and stress, he began to stop himself from eating, rather than expecting something external to stop him. He had his surgery, and now has kept the weight off for over three years. The surgery will work short term, but it will not work long term without the patient also learning to use the mind. If you are looking for something, other than you, to stop you from eating, weight loss will be short lived. For Alberto, it will mean he must focus on diet and exercise for the rest of his life. But this time he now has the psychological tools to help him accomplish his goals.

start eating more than they should, which in turn stretches out the pouch.

Again, the best action is to contact a psychologist as soon as possible, before irreversible damage has been done to the pouch. With serious effort, you can learn to be in control of your eating behavior.

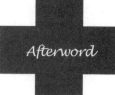

With the decision to have bariatric surgery, you have also decided to take back control of your health. After weight loss, your future looks brighter, your health will improve, and your choices in life increase. Hopefully, the information in this book will help you with the daunting task of maintaining your weight loss for life. For some patients, maintenance will be a breeze and habits will become automatic. For others, it will be a lifelong struggle, but one that can be won. Remember to always ask for help if you need it. The quest for a healthy life will never end, but the benefits and rewards definitely "outweigh" the challenge.

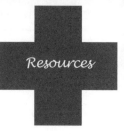
Resources

Academy for Eating Disorders. 6728 Old McLean
Village Drive, McLean, VA 22101
www.aedweb.org.

Adami GF, Meneghelli A, Bressani A, Scopinaro, N.
Body image in obese patients before and after
stable weight reduction following bariatric
surgery. *Journal of Psychosomatic Research*
1999;46(3):275–81.

Adolfsson B, Andersson I, Elofsson S, et al. Locus of
control and weight reduction. *Patient
Education and Counseling* 2005;56(1):55–61.

American College of Sports Medicine. (ACSM)
P.O. Box,1440, Indianapolis, IN 46206
www.acsm.org/index.asp.

American Psychiatric Association. *Diagnostic and
Statistical Manual on Mental Disorders,
Fourth Edition, Text Revision.* Washington
DC: American Psychiatric Publishing, Inc., 2000.

American Society for Bariatric Surgery. 100 S.W. 75th
St. Suite 201. Gainesville, FL 32607.
www.asbs.org.

Armitage A. Motivating overweight adults to lose weight. *Clinical Excellence for Nurse Practitioners* 2003;7(4):92–8.

Armstrong CA, Sallis JF, Hovell M, Hofsetter CR. Stages of change, self-efficacy, and the adoption of vigorous exercise: A prospective analysis. *Journal of Sport & Exercise Psychology* 1993;15:390–402.

Baile WF, Engel BT. A behavioral strategy or promoting treatment compliance following myocardial infarction. *Psychosomatic Medicine* 1978;40:413–19.

Baker RC, Kirschenbaum DS. Weight control during the holidays: Highly consistent self-monitoring as a potentially useful coping mechanism. *Health Psychology* 1998;17(4).

Ball K, Lee C. Psychological stress, coping, and symptoms of disordered eating in a community sample of young Australian women. *International Journal of Eating Disorders* 2002;31(1):71–81.

Bandrua A, Walters RH. *Social Learning and Personality Development.* New York: Holt, Rinehart, and Winston, 1963.

Bandura A, Simon KM. The role of proximal intentions in self-regulation of refractory behavior. *Cognitive Therapy and Research* 1977;1:177–93.

Bandura A. Self-efficacy: Toward a unifying theory of behavioral change. *Psychological Review* 1977;84:191–215.

Beck JS. *Cognitive Therapy: Basics and Beyond.* New York: Guilford Press, 1995.

Benotti PN, Forse RA. The role of gastric surgery in the multidisciplinary management of severe obesity. *The American Journal of Surgery* 1995;169:361–7.

Bittinger JN, Smith JE. Mediating and moderating effects of stress perception and situational coping responses in women with disordered eating. *Eating Behaviors* 2003;4(1):89–1–6.

Blaine BE, DiBlasi DM, Connor JM. The effect of weight loss on perceptions of weight controllability: Implications for prejudice against overweight people. *Journal of Applied Biobehavioral Research* 2002;7(1):44–56.

Blaine B, Williams Z. Belief in the controllability of weight and attributions to prejudice against heavyweight women. *Sex Roles* 2004;51(1–2):79–84.

Boon B, Stroebe W, Schut H. Food for thought: Cognitive regulation of food intake. *British Journal of Health Psychology* 1998;3:27–40.

Booth DA, Blair AJ, Lewis VJ, Baek SH. Patterns of eating and movement that best maintain reduction in overweight. *Appetite* 2004;43(3):277–83.

Brownell KD. Behavioral medicine. In: Franks CM, Wilson GT, Kendall P, Brownell KD (eds). *Annual Review of Behavior Therapy: Theory and Practice. Volume Eight.* New York: Guildford Press, 1982.

Brownell KD, Foreyt JP (eds). *The Handbook of Eating Disorders. Physiology, Psychology and Treatment of Obesity, Anorexia, and Bulimia.* New York: Basic Books, HarperCollins Publishers, 1986.

Brownell KD. *The LEARN Program for Weight Control.* Dallas, TX: Brownell & Hager, 1989.

Byrne SM. Psychological aspects of weight maintenance and relapse in obesity. *Journal of Psychosomatic Research* 2002;53(5):1029–36.

Byrne S, Cooper Z, Fairburn C. Weight maintenance and relapse in obesity: A qualitative study. *International Journal of Obesity and Related Metabolic Disorders* 2003;27(8):955–62.

Byrne SM, Cooper Z, Fairburn CG. Psychological predictors of weight regain in obesity. *Behaviour Research and Therapy* 2004;42(11):1341–56.

Camerini G, Adami GF, Marinari G, et al. Satiety after vertical banded gastroplasty. *Eating and Weight Disorders* 2003;8(1):80–3.

Carels RA, Douglass OM, Cacciapaglia HM, O'Brien WH. An ecological momentary assessment of relapse crises in dieting. *Journal of Consulting & Clinical Psychology* 2004;72(2):341–8.

Castellani W, Ianni L, Ricca V, et al. Adherence to structured physical exercise in overweight and obese: A review of psychological models. *Eating and Weight Disorders* 2003;8(1):1–11.

Castelnuovo-Tedesco P, Douglas S. Studies of superobesity II. Psychiatric appraisal of jejuno-ileal bypass surgery. *American Journal of Psychiatry* 1976;133(1):26–31.

Claiborn J, Pedrick CT. *The Habit Change Workbook: How to Break Bad Habits and Form Good Ones.* Oakland, CA: New Harbinger Publications, Inc., 2001.

Cossrow NHF, Jeffery RW, McGuire MT. Understanding weight stigmatization: A focus group study. *Journal of Nutrition Education* 2001;33(4):208–14.

Davis M, Eshelman E, McKay M. *The Relaxation and Stress Reduction Workbook, Fifth Edition.* Oakland, CA: New Harbinger Publications, Inc., 2000.

Delin CR, Anderson PG. A preliminary comparison of the psychological impact of laparoscopic gastric banding and gastric bypass surgery for morbid obesity. *Obesity Surgery* 1999;9:155–60.

Dittman M. Weighing in on fat bias. *Monitor on Psychology.* American Psychological Association, 2004;35(1).

Dohm FA, Beattie JA, Aibel C, Striegel-Moore RH. Factors differentiating women and men who successfully maintain weight loss from women and men who do not. *Journal of Clinical Psychology* 2001;57(1):105–17.

Drapkin RG, Wing RR, Shiffman S. Responses to hypothetical high risk situations: Do they predict weight loss in a behavioral treatment program or the context of dietary lapses? *Health Psychology* 1995;14(5):427.

Dymek MP, Le Grange D, Neven K, Alverdy J. Quality of life and psychosocial adjustment in patients after roux-en-y gastric bypass: A brief report. *Obesity Surgery* 2004;11(1):32–9.

Epstein L, Cluss P. A behavioral medicine perspective on adherence to long-term medical regimens. *Journal of Consulting and Clinical Psychology* 1982;50:950–71.

Eton DT. Social support and its relation to weight control: An empirical analysis. *Dissertation Abstracts International: Section B—The Sciences & Engineering* 1999;59(11-B):6115.

Fobi MAL. Surgical treatment of obesity: A review. *Journal of the National Medical Association* 2004;96(1):61–75.

Foreyt JP, Goodrick GK. Attributes of successful approaches to weight loss and control. *Applied and Preventive Psychology* 1994;3(4):209–15.

Foreyt JP, Goodrick GK. Factors common to successful therapy for the obese patient. *Medicine and Science in Sports and Exercise* 1991;23(3):292–7.

Foster GD, Wadden TA, Vogt RA. Body image in obese women before, during, and after weight loss treatment. *Health Psychology* 1997;16(3).

Freeman LM, Gil KM. Daily stress, coping, and dietary restraint in binge eating. *International Journal of Eating Disorders* 2004;36(2):204–12.

Gauron EF. *Mental Training for Peak Performance.* Lansing, NY: Sport Science Associates, 1984.

Gauvin L. An experiential perspective on the motivational features of exercise and lifestyle. *Canadian Journal of Sport Sciences* 1990;15:51–8.

Glinski J, Wetzler S, Goodman E. The psychology of gastric bypass surgery. *Obesity Surgery* 2001;11:581–8.

Golay A, Buclin S, Ybarra J, et al. New interdisciplinary cognitive-behavioural-nutritional approach to obesity treatment: A 5-year follow-up study. *Eating and Weight Disorders* 2004;9(1):29–34.

Gorin AA, Phelan S, Hill JO, Wing RR. Medical triggers are associated with better short- and long-term weight outcomes. *Preventive Medicine: An International Journal Devoted to Practice and Theory* 2004;39(3).

Gorin AA, Phenlan S, Wing RR, Hill JO. Promoting long-term weight control: Does dieting consistency matter? *International Journal of Obesity and Related Metabolic Disorders* 2004;28(2):278–81.

Green CG, Wing RR. Stress-induced eating. *Psychological Bulletin* 1994;115(3).

Grilo CM, Shiffman S, Wing R. Relapse crises and coping among dieters. *Journal of Consulting and Clinical Psychology* 1989;57(4):488–95.

Grilo CM, Shiffman S. Longitudinal investigation of the abstinence violation effect in binge eating. *Journal of Consulting and Clinical Psychology* 1994;62(3):611–19.

Grilo M. The assessment and treatment of binge eating disorders. *Journal of Practical Psychiatry and Behavioral Health* 1998;4:191–201.

Guisado JA, Vaz FJ, Lopez-Ibor MI, et al. Gastric surgery and restraint from food as triggering factors of eating disorders in morbid obesity. *International Journal of Eating Disorders* 2002;31(1):97–100.

Guisado JA, Vaz FJ, Alarcon J, et al. Psychopathological status and interpersonal functioning following weight loss in morbidly obese patients undergoing bariatric surgery. *Obesity Surgery* 2004;12(6):835–40.

Guisado JA, Vaz FJ. Psychopathological differences between morbidly obese binge eaters and non-binge eaters after bariatric surgery. *Eating and Weight Disorders* 2003;8(4):315–18.

Hafner RJ, Rogers J, and Watts JM. Psychological status before and after gastric restriction as predictors of weight loss in the morbidly obese. *Journal of Psychosomatic Research* 1990;34(3):295–302.

Harris DV, Harris BL. *The Athlete's Guide to Sport Psychology: Mental Training for Physical People.* New York: Leisure Press, 1984.

Head S, Brookhart A. Lifestyle modification and relapse prevention training during treatment for weight loss. *Behavior Therapy* 1997;28(2):307–21.

Hergenhahn BR, Olson MH. *An Introduction to Theories of Learning, Sixth Edition.* Upper Saddle River, NJ: Prentice Hall, 2001.

Hitchcock P, Pugh JA. Management of overweight and obese adults. *British Medical Journal* 2002;325:757–61.

Hsu LKG, Benotti PN, Dwyer J, et al. Nonsurgical factors that influence the outcome of bariatric surgery: A review. *Psychosomatic Medicine* 1998;60(3):338–46.

Jacobson E. The origins and development of progressive relaxation. *Journal of Behavior Therapy & Experimental Psychiatry* 1977;8(2):119–23.

Jacobson E. *Progressive Relaxation.* Chicago, IL: University of Chicago Press, 1938.

Jakicic JM, Clark K, Coleman E, et al. Appropriate intervention strategies for weight loss and prevention of weight regain for adults. *Medicine and Science in Sports and Exercise* 2001;33(12):2145–56.

Janis IL, Mann L. *Decision Making: A Psychological Analysis of Conflict, Choice and Commitment.* New York: Free Press, 1977.

Kalarchian MA, Terence WG, Brolin RE, Bradley L. Binge eating in bariatric surgery patients. *International Journal of Eating Disorders* 1998;23(1):89–92.

Kalarchian MA, Marcus MD. Management of the bariatric surgery patient: Is there a role for the cognitive behavior therapist? *Cognitive and Behavioral Practice* 2003;10:112–19.

King TK, Clark MM, Pera V. History of sexual abuse and obesity treatment outcome. *Addictive Behaviors* 1996;21(3):283–90.

Kirschenbaum DS, Dykman BM. Disinhibited eating by resourceful restrained eaters. *Journal of Abnormal Psychology* 1991;100(2):227–30.

Korotitsch WJ, Nelson-Gray RO. An overview of self-monitoring research in assessment and treatment. *Psychological Assessment* 1999;11(4):415.

Kraft AM. Weight loss and depression. *American Journal of Psychiatry* 1991;148(7):947–8.

Kumar N, Singh JG. A study of surgical stress among female patients. *Journal of Personality and Clinical Studies* 2001;17(2);100–7.

Laitinen J, Ek E, Sovio U. Stress-related eating and drinking behavior and body mass index as predictors of this behavior. *Preventative Medicine: An International Journal Devoted to Practice and Theory* 2002;34(1).

Larimer JE, Palmer RS, Marlatt GA. Relapse prevention: An overview of Marlatt's cognitive-behavioral model. *Alcohol Research and Health* 1999;23(2):151–60.

Lewis VJ, Blair AJ, Booth DA. Outcome of group therapy for body-image emotionality and weight-control self-efficacy. *Behavioural Psychotherapy* 1992;20:155–65.

Locke EA, Lathan GP. *A Theory of Goal Setting and Task Performance.* Englewood Cliffs, NJ: Prentice Hall, 1990.

Logue AW. Evolutionary theory and the psychology of eating (1998). Access date: March 28, 2005. Available at: darwin.baruch.cuny.edu/faculty/LogueA.html.

Marcoux BC, Trenkner LL, Rosenstock IM. Social networks and social support in weight loss. *Patient Education and Counseling* 1990;15(3):229–38.

Marcus JD, Elkins GR. Development of a model for a structured support group for patients following bariatric surgery. *Obesity Surgery* 2004;14:103–6.

Marcus JD, Elkins GR. Laparoscopic adjustable gastric band: Do support groups add to the weight loss? *Obesity Surgery* 2004;14(8):1139–40.

Marlatt GA, Gordon J. *Relapse Prevention: Maintenance Strategies in Addictive Behavior Change.* New York: Guilford Press, 1985.

Martin JE, Dubbert PM, Katell AD, et al. Behavior control of exercise in sedentary adults: Studies 1–6. *Journal of Consulting and Clinical Psychology* 1984;52:795–811.

McElroy SL, Kotwal R, Shishuka M, et al. Are mood disorders and obesity related? A review for the mental health profession. *Journal of Clinical Psychiatry* 2004;65(5):634–51.

McGuire MT, Wing RR, Klem ML, et al. What predicts weight regain in a group of successful weight losers. *Journal of Consulting & Clinical Psychology* 1999;67(3).

Meichenbaum D. *Cognitive-Behavior Modification.* New York: Plenum, 1977.

Miller CT, Rothblum ED, Felicio D, Brand P. Compensating for stigma: Obese and nonobese women's reactions to being visible. *Personality and Social Psychology Bulletin* 1995;21(10):1093–106.

Mitchell JE, deZwan M (eds). *Bariatric Surgery: A Guide for Mental Health Professionals.* New York, NY: Routledge, 2005.

Mooney JP, Burling TA, Hartman WM, Brenner-Liss D. The abstinence violation effect and very low calorie diet success. *Addictive Behaviors* 1992;17(4):319–24.

Musher-Eizenman DR, Holub SC, Miller AB, et al. Body size stigmatization in preschool children: The role of control in attributions. *Journal of Pediatric Psychology* 2004;29(8):613–20.

Myers AW, Schleser RA. A cognitive-behavioral intervention for improving basketball performance. *Journal of Sport Psychology* 1980;3:69–73.

National Eating Disorder Association. 603 Stewart Street, Suite 803, Seattle, WA 98101 www.nationaleatingdisorders.org.

National Institute of Mental Health. 6001 Executive Blvd. Room 8184, Bethesda, MD 20892 www.nimh.nih.gov.

National Strength and Conditioning Association. 1955 N. Union Blvd., Colorado Springs, CO 80909. www.nsca-lift.org.

Nejad LM, Wertheim EH, Greenwood KM. Predicted dieting behavior by using, modifying, and extending the theory of planned behavior. *Journal of Applied Social Psychology* 2004;34(10):2099–131.

Nickels R, Sayeed S, Sax HC. Predicting success after gastric bypass: The role of psychosocial and behavioral factors. *Surgery* 2003;134(4):555–63.

O'Connor DB, O'Connor RC. Perceived changes in food intake in response to stress: The role of conscientiousness. *Stress and Health: Journal of the International Society for the Investigation of Stress* 2004;20(5):279–91.

Ogden J, Whyman C. The effect of repeated weighing on psychological state. *European Eating Disorders Review* 1997;5(2):121–30.

Ogden J, Wardle J. Control of eating and attributional style. *British Journal of Clinical Psychology* 1990;29(4):445–6.

Pavlov IP. *Conditioned Reflexes.* London: Oxford University Press, 1927.

Perri MG, Martin AD, Leermakers EA, et al. Effects of group versus home based exercise in the treatment of obesity. *Journal of Consulting and Clinical Psychology* 1997;65(2).

Perri MG, Nezu AM, McKelvey WF, Shermer RL. Relapse prevention training and problem-solving therapy in the long-term management of obesity. *Journal of Consulting and Clinical Psychology* 2001;69(4):722.

Polivy J, Herman CP, McFarlane T. Effects of anxiety on eating: Does palatability moderate distress-induced overeating in dieters? *Journal of Abnormal Psychology* 1994;103(30):505–10.

Porter LC, Wampler RS. Adjustment to rapid weight loss. *Families, Systems, and Health* 2000;18(1):35–54.

President's Council on Physical Fitness and Sports. Dept. W, 200 Independence Ave, SW, Room 738-H. Washington, DC 20201 www.fitness.gov.

Prochaska JO, DiClemente CC. Transtheoretical therapy: Toward a more integrative model of change. *Psychotherapy: Theory, Research and Practice* 1982;19:276–88.

Raglin JS. Exercise and mental health: Beneficial and detrimental effects. *Sports Medicine* 1990;9:323–9.

Rich LE. Along with increased surgery, a growing need for support. American Psychological Association: *Monitor on Psychology* 2004;35(1).

Rosenstock IM. Historical origins of the health belief model. *Health Education Monographs* 1966;2:323–9.

Saunders R, Johnson L, Teschner J. Prevalence of eating disorders among bariatric surgery patients. *Eating Disorders: The Journal of Treatment & Prevention* 1998;6(4):309–17.

Saunders R. Compulsive eating and gastric bypass surgery: What does hunger have to do with it? *Obesity Surgery* 2001;11:757–61.

Saunders R. "Grazing:" A high-risk behavior. *Obesity Surgery* 2004;14:98–102.

Schwartz MB, Brownell KD. Obesity and body image. *Body Image* 2003;1:43–56.

Sjostrom L, Lindroos A, Peltonen M, et al. Lifestyle, diabetes, and cardiovascular risk factors 10 years after bariatric surgery. *New England Journal of Medicine* 2004;351(26):2683–93.

Skinner BF. *Science and Human Behavior.* New York: Macmillan, 1953.

Solomon CG, Dluhy RG. Bariatric surgery: Quick fix or long term solution? *New England Journal of Medicine* 2004;351(26):2751–3.

Stunkard AJ, Faith MS, Allison KC. Depression and obesity. *Biological Psychiatry* 2003;54(3):330–7.

Wadden TA, Stunkard AJ (eds). *Handbook of Obesity Treatment.* New York, NY, Guilford Press, 2002.

Wadden TA, Sarwer DB, Womble LG, et al. Psychosocial aspects of obesity and obesity surgery. *Obesity Surgery* 2001;81(5):1001–24.

Wallis DJ, Hetherington MM. Stress and eating: The effects of ego-threat and cognitive demand on food intake in restrained and emotional eaters. *Appetite* 2004;43:39–46.

Ward A, Mann T. Don't mind if I do: Disinhibited eating under cognitive load. *Journal of Personality and Social Psychology* 2000;78(4).

Weinberg RS, Weigand D. Goal setting in sport and exercise. A reaction to Locke. *Journal of Sport & Exercise Psychology* 1993;15:88–95.

Williams P, Lord S. Predictors of adherence to a structured exercise program for older women. *Psychology and Aging* 1995;10(4).

Wooley SC, Wooley OW, Dyrenforth SR. Theoretical, practical, and social issues in behavioral treatments of obesity. *Journal of Applied Behavior Analysis* 1979;12:3–25.

Yalom ID. *Theory and Practice of Group Psychotherapy.* New York: BasicBooks. A Division of HarperCollins Publishers, Inc., 1995.

Other resources available from

Matrix Medical Communications

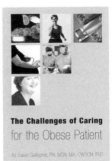

NOTES

NOTES

NOTES